An Atlas of
INFANT POLYSOMNOGRAPHY

THE ENCYCLOPEDIA OF VISUAL MEDICINE SERIES

An Atlas of
INFANT POLYSOMNOGRAPHY

David H. Crowell, PhD
and the CHIME Study Group

The Parthenon Publishing Group
International Publishers in Medicine, Science & Technology

A CRC PRESS COMPANY

BOCA RATON   LONDON   NEW YORK   WASHINGTON, D.C.

Published in the USA by
The Parthenon Publishing Group
345 Park Avenue South, 10th Floor
New York
NY 10010
USA

Published in the UK and Europe by
The Parthenon Publishing Group
23–25 Blades Court
Deodar Road
London SW15 2NU
UK

Library of Congress Cataloging-in-Publication Data
Data available on request

British Library Cataloguing in Publication Data
Crowell, David H. (David Harrison), 1919-
   An atlas of infant polysomnography. - (The encyclopedia of visual medicine series)
   1. Polysomnography 2. Sleep disorders in children 3. Infants -
   Sleep
   I. Title II. CHIME Study Group
   618.9'28498

ISBN 1-84214-194-5

First published in 2003

Composition by The Parthenon Publishing Group
Printed and bound by Bookcraft (Bath) Ltd., Midsomer Norton, UK

Contents

List of authors   7

Foreword   9

Acknowledgements   11

1   Introduction   15

2   Basics of physiological signal acquisition and processing for infant polysomnography   19

3   Infant polysomnography recording procedures   39

4   Infant polysomnography scoring procedures   63

Appendix

A   Caregiver education   139

B   Infant polysomnography checklist   141

C   Modification of the International 10–20 system measurements for infant polysomnography   145

D   Documentation   146

E   Quality review   148

F   Apnea/hypopnea measurement   149

G   Elimination of spurious and artifactual signals   151

Glossary   153

Index   163

List of authors

David H. Crowell, PhD
Associate Director
Sleep Disorders Center of the Pacific
Straub Clinic & Hospital
Honolulu, Hawaii 96813

and

Clinical Professor of Pediatrics
Department of Pediatrics
John A. Burns School of Medicine
University of Hawaii at Manoa
Honolulu, Hawaii 96822

Linda E. Kapuniai, DrPH
Clinical Associate
Sleep Disorders Center of the Pacific
Straub Clinic & Hospital
Honolulu, Hawaii 96813

and

Adjunct Assistant Professor of Pediatrics
Department of Pediatrics
John A. Burns School of Medicine
University of Hawaii at Manoa
Honolulu, Hawaii 96822

Toke T. Hoppenbrouwers, PhD
Clinical Professor of Pediatrics
Division of Neonatology
Keck School of Medicine, University of Southern
 California
Women's and Children's Hospital
Los Angeles, California 90033

Lee J. Brooks, MD
Pediatric Pulmonologist
The Children's Hospital of Philadelphia
Philadelphia, Pennsylvania 19104

and

Clinical Associate Professor of Pediatrics
University of Pennsylvania
Philadelphia, Pennsylvania

Michael R. Neuman, PhD, MD
Professor of Biomedical Engineering and Herff Chair
 of Excellence
Joint Graduate Program in Biomedical Engineering
The University of Memphis and The University of
 Tennessee Health Science Center
Memphis, Tennessee 38152

and

Professor, Department of Pediatrics
The University of Tennessee Health Science Center
Memphis, Tennessee

Sally L. Davidson Ward, MD
Associate Professor of Pediatrics
Division of Pediatric Pulmonology
Keck School of Medicine, University of Southern
 California
Childrens Hospital of Los Angeles
Los Angeles, California 90027

Carl E. Hunt, MD
Director, National Sleep Center on Sleep Disorders
    Research
National Heart, Lung and Blood Institute
Bethesda, Maryland 20892

and

Adjunct Professor of Pediatrics
Uniformed Services University of the Health
    Sciences
Bethesda, Maryland

Debra E. Weese-Mayer, MD
Director, Pediatric Respiratory Medicine
Rush Children's Hospital at Rush-Presbyterian-St.
    Luke's Medical Center
Chicago, Illinois 60612

and

Professor of Pediatrics
Rush University
Chicago, Illinois

Michael J. Corwin, MD
Co-Director, Massachusetts Center for SIDS
Boston Medical Center
Boston, Massachusetts 02118

and

Associate Professor of Pediatrics and Epidemiology
Boston University Schools of Medicine and Public
    Health
Boston, Massachusetts

Mark Peucker
Vice President of Information Technology
Carestat
180 Wells Avenue
Newton, Massachusetts 02459

George Lister, MD
Director, Pediatric Intensive Care Unit
Yale–New Haven Children's Hospital
New Haven, Connecticut

and

Professor of Pediatrics and Anesthesiology
Yale University, School of Medicine
New Haven, Connecticut

Larry R. Tinsley, MD
Department of Neonatology
Pomona Medical Center
Pediatric Critical Care Medical Group/Pediatric
    Management Group
Childrens Hospital of Los Angeles
Los Angeles, California 90027

Jean M. Silvestri, MD
Director, Center for Disorders of Respiratory
    Control
Rush Children's Hospital at Rush-Presbyterian-St.
    Luke's Medical Center
Chicago, Illinois 60612

and

Associate Professor of Pediatrics
Rush University
Chicago, Illinois

Marian Willinger, PhD
Special Assistant for SIDS
Pregnancy and Perinatology Branch
Center for Research for Mothers and Children
National Institute of Child Health and Human
    Development
Bethesda, Maryland 20892

James W. Pearce, MD
Director, Sleep Disorders Center of the Pacific
Straub Clinic & Hospital
Honolulu, Hawaii 96813

and

Associate Professor
Department of Neurology
John A. Burns School of Medicine
University of Hawaii at Manoa
Honolulu, Hawaii 96822

Foreword

Long-term sleep recording of infants gives us a great deal of information about the functioning of the brainstem and related nuclei. These include regulation of respiration, heart rate, sleep and waking, eye movements, and vocalizations, such as crying and other sounds. These are all fundamental functions for survival. When we first started making such recordings, each investigator used a somewhat different recording technique. This made it very difficult to compare data obtained accurately so that we could determine what to consider deviant from normal sleep and arousal development. Gradually, investigators began to try to standardize basic recording techniques and terminology for interpretation of the recorded data. The enormous value of the CHIME's Atlas cannot be overestimated. This group has done a great service for all of us by preparing this very detailed recording Atlas. It will profoundly increase the value of all infant sleep data collected in the future.

For those of us who began studying infant sleep a number of years ago there were no guidelines. Most of our help came from animal sleep studies carried out by neurophysiologists and their technicians. Drs Hoppenbrouwers and Crowell were among those who began to bring some order to this field of investigation and I was fortunate enough to be in touch with them early on. The CHIME groups are currently active in long-term sleep recording and have been able to contribute the latest available electronic and behavioral information. I don't think it is possible to overestimate the value of the Atlas.

Arthur H. Parmelee, Jr., MD

*Professor of Pediatrics, Emeritus, School of Medicine,
University of California, Los Angeles*

Acknowledgements

The Collaborative Home Infant Monitoring Evaluation (CHIME) study developed a nocturnal polysomnography protocol and procedures that serve as the basis for the majority of the polysomnographic methodology and examples in this Atlas. Untold hours of effort on the part of CHIME investigators and other personnel and many nights of staying awake for the polysomnography technicians contributed to the successful outcomes presented. The procedures described herein are the result of years of experience and training on the part of the members of the CHIME PSG committee (DHC, TTH, LJB, SLDW, MRN). To recognize the collaborative efforts of the CHIME Study Group, the group members and their affiliations during the CHIME study are listed below.

The CHIME study was supported by NICHD HD: 29067, 29071, 28971, 29073, 29060, 29056 and 34625. The participants in the CHIME Study Group include:

(*Principal Investigator, **Study Coordinator)

CLINICAL SITES

Department of Pediatrics, Case Western Reserve University School of Medicine, Cleveland, OH

MetroHealth Medical Center
Terry M. Baird*

Rainbow Babies and Children's Hospital
Richard J. Martin
Lee J. Brooks
Roberta O'Bell**

Department of Pediatrics, Medical College of Ohio, Toledo Hospital and St. Vincent Mercy Medical Center, Toledo, OH
Carl E. Hunt*
David R. Hufford
Mary Ann Oess**

Department of Pediatrics, Division of Respiratory Medicine, Rush Medical College of Rush University, Chicago, IL
Rush Children's Hospital at Rush-Presbyterian-St. Luke's Medical Center
Debra E. Weese-Mayer*
Jean M. Silvestri
Sheilah M. Smok-Pearsall**

Department of Pediatrics, John A. Burns School of Medicine, University of Hawaii at Manoa, Honolulu, HI

Kapi'olani Medical Center for Women and Children
David H. Crowell*
Larry R. Tinsley
Linda E. Kapuniai**

Department of Pediatrics and Neonatology, USC School of Medicine, Los Angeles, CA

Los Angeles County & USC Medical Center, Women's and Children's Hospital and Good Samaritan Hospital
Toke T. Hoppenbrouwers*
Rangasamy Ramanathan
Paula Palmer**

Childrens Hospital Los Angeles
Thomas G. Keens
Sally L. Davidson Ward
Daisy B. Bolduc, Technical Coordinator

CLINICAL TRIALS OPERATIONS CENTER

Department of Obstetrics and Gynecology, Case Western University School of Medicine and MetroHealth Medical Center, Cleveland, OH
Michael R. Neuman*
Rebecca S. Mendenhall**

DATA COORDINATING AND ANALYSIS CENTER

Departments of Pediatrics and Epidemiology and Biostatistics, Boston University Schools of Medicine and Public Health, Boston, MA
Michael J. Corwin*
Theodore Colton
Sharon M. Bak**
Mark Peucker, Technical Coordinator
Howard Golub, Physiologic Data Biostatistician
Susan C. Schafer, Clinical Trials Coordinator

STEERING COMMITTEE CHAIRMAN

Department of Pediatrics, Yale University School of Medicine, New Haven, CT
George Lister

NATIONAL INSTITUTES OF HEALTH (NIH)

Pregnancy and Perinatology Branch, Center for Research for Mothers and Children, National Institute of Child Health and Human Development (NICHD), NIH, Bethesda, MD
Marian Willinger

The CHIME study recognizes the contributions of Healthdyne, Inc., Marietta, GA (now Respironics, Inc.) and Non-Invasive Monitoring Systems (NIMS), Miami, FL. The ALICE 3™ data acquisition and analysis systems used by all CHIME sites included a 486/33 IBM computer, 20-inch monitor and optical disk storage media with software versions 1.17 or 1.19. For the CHIME protocol, the CHIME home monitor (NIMS) was interfaced with ALICE 3™ to record cardiorespiratory variables and SaO_2.

The authors want to recognize the following institutions and individuals that facilitated the preparation of the manuscript: Kapiʻolani Medical Center for Women & Children, Honolulu, Hawaii; Straub Clinic & Hospital, Honolulu, Hawaii; John A. Burns School of Medicine, University of Hawaii at Manoa, Honolulu, Hawaii.

Supportive individuals at these institutions were: (1) Dew-Anne Langcaon, Executive Vice-President; Dexter Seto, MD, Director of Research and Harry F. Skidmore, Director, Kapiʻolani Health Research Institute; Jana Hall, Executive Director, Hawaii Pacific Health Research Institute; (2) Edwin Cadman, MD, Dean of the John A. Burns School of Medicine, University of Hawaii, Honolulu, Hawaii; (3) Billie Ikeda, Graphic Media Design, Center for Instructional Support, Office of Faculty Development and Academic Support, University of Hawaii, Honolulu, Hawaii; (4) Karen Mayeda, Straub Clinic & Hospital, photography; and (5) Kristi Sakamoto and James Hokama, computer specialists.

I

Introduction

Infant polysomnography (IPSG) holds great promise for the study of sleep and breathing disorders, the functional integrity of the developing brain and early cardiorespiratory functioning. For IPSG to be most useful, results from different studies need to be derived from comparable techniques in data acquisition and measurement[1]. Although guidelines and standards have been developed[2-8], there is no one source for IPSG applied to infants over time, starting with pre-terms and continuing past 6 months post-term. Polysomnography, or the simultaneous recording of multiple physiological variables during sleep, is considered the gold standard for recording sleep and sleep-related events. Clinicians and investigators, however, have different views on the duration, timing and content of physiological monitoring in infants. This Atlas offers one view by incorporating procedures for recording and scoring sleep and sleep-related events in this age group.

HISTORICAL VIEW

Early studies relied on direct observations of sleeping infants and rudimentary physiological monitoring[9-14]. The impetus for physiological monitoring of sleep in young infants came from the observation of rapid eye movements (REMs) by Aserinsky and Kleitman[15,16]. Concepts such as the basic rest activity cycle[17] and a desire to investigate basic central nervous system activity stimulated a plethora of infant sleep studies in the 1960s and 1970s[11,18-22]. With advances in recording technology, many clinicians and investigators developed protocols for infant sleep studies (see above) and a standardized protocol for full-term newborns was published by

Anders and colleagues in 1971[2]. Indications and standards for cardiopulmonary sleep studies in children were developed by the American Thoracic Society in 1996[3] and promulgated by the American Academy of Pediatrics in 2002[23,24].

As has been the case in the development of adult polysomnography, infant sleep studies have evolved and systems for data acquisition and analysis have varied depending on the purposes and resources available to scientists and clinicians. Over the last 10 years rapid developments in computer technology and accessibility have offered alternatives that range from traditional mechanical analog recorders such as polygraphs to digital computer data acquisition, storage and analysis systems. This Atlas presents procedures in terms that can be used with both analog polygraphs and computerized systems.

During the same period that IPSG was coming of age, concern for preventing sudden infant death syndrome (SIDS) was gaining support. The Consensus Conference on Infantile Apnea and Home Monitoring[25] outlined the need for increased efforts to understand the physiological, behavioral and developmental aspects of SIDS, including a focus on factors associated with sleep state. Responding to this call for action, in 1991 the National Institute of Child Health and Human Development of the USA initiated a multicenter nationwide research project, the Collaborative Home Infant Monitoring Evaluation (CHIME). Although the primary focus of CHIME was home cardiorespiratory monitoring, the protocol recognized the importance of including nocturnal IPSG in order to:

(1) Identify PSG patterns associated with clinically important events (severe apnea, bradycardia and oxygen saturation) documented by home monitoring. These patterns and events included sleep architecture, central and obstructive sleep apnea and other respiratory disturbances, heart rate, and oxygen saturation.

(2) Determine whether abnormal maturation of the autonomic and central nervous systems as measured by electroencephalograph (EEG) patterns or vagal tone are precursors of clinically important events.

(3) Validate the accuracy of the CHIME home monitor by using it during overnight IPSGs.

CHIME required that the IPSGs be nocturnal because the long duration offered the opportunity to record sleep and cardiorespiratory variables over a substantial period of time, and the nocturnal time-frame included the early morning hours thought to be associated with increased risk for SIDS[26].

CHIME IPSG recordings were acquired under standardized conditions at several clinical sites (see Acknowledgements). To achieve this a detailed procedural manual was developed, evaluated and implemented at all sites. The procedures tested in the CHIME study form the basis of the recommendations in this Atlas. The CHIME database includes what were then state-of-the-art physiological recordings in the sleep laboratory environment on 415 infants with gestational ages ranging from 26 to 41 weeks and conceptional ages ranging from 34 to 62 weeks. There were four CHIME study groups including: healthy term infants, infants who were born prematurely, siblings of SIDS victims, and infants who had experienced an idiopathic apparent life-threatening event or apnea of infancy. Infants were excluded from the study if they had: current caregiver illicit drug use, language barrier, no telephone in the home, current pneumonia, home treatment with bronchodilators, diuretics, steroids, respiratory stimulants other than methylxanthines, continuous oxygen need, congenital heart disease other than asymptomatic patent ductus arteriosus, atrioseptal defect, ventriculoseptal defect, brain anomalies, ventriculo-peritoneal shunt, home anticonvulsant therapy, congenital and chromosomal anomalies, and inborn errors of metabolism.

The goal of this Atlas is to offer researchers and clinicians the benefit of the CHIME experience with nocturnal IPSG in this age group and to demonstrate that high-quality recordings of sleep and cardiorespiratory variables can be obtained, measured and analyzed. Infant sleep data can be accumulated to address multiple issues related to ontogeny and normal development. This Atlas is a fundamental resource for sleep researchers who work with infants from 35 weeks' conceptional age to 6 months post-term.

There are well-recognized limitations and special difficulties associated with conducting long-duration recordings in infants in the age range covered here. For example, there are necessary interventions and disruptions associated with comforting, feeding and diaper changing. The effects of a new sleep environment and dealing with multiple sensors, particularly those on the head and face, are difficult to estimate. Nevertheless, this Atlas is unique in terms of the age range addressed and the depth of the graphic illustrations of IPSG parameters, sleep states and the transition to sleep stages, as well as other physiological events that occur during sleep.

The contents of this Atlas encompass fundamentals of polysomnography that would be essential to a pediatric sleep laboratory. Then, using examples from the CHIME experience, illustrations are presented for data acquisition, recording and monitoring considerations, sleep state and stage definitions, and cardiorespiratory patterns and events. In many clinical settings, an abbreviated recording, usually referred to as a pneumogram or sleep study, is used to monitor cardiorespiratory signals during a nap, overnight or for a prolonged (12–24 h) period. These sleep studies typically record some combination of the electrocardiogram (ECG), respiratory effort and possibly airflow, and in some cases pulse oximetry; what is not included are the parameters that define sleep and wake states. This Atlas focuses on:

• PSG in contrast to a more limited study

• Directions on how to achieve optimal PSG results in very young infants

• Reliable techniques for scoring sleep and events

• Waveform examples

A typical array of recording parameters is the same for infants as for older children and adults and will include, but not be limited to, the following:

- The electroencephalogram (EEG)

- The electrooculogram (EOG)

- The electromyogram (EMG)

- The electrocardiogram (ECG)

- Nasal and possibly oral airflow

- Respiratory effort or motion from the rib cage and abdomen

- Pulse oximetry, including the pulse waveform

- Sleep position from direct observations and/or monitoring

- Body movements

In addition to these signals, IPSG requires special attention not only to the recording environment and behavioral documentation, but also to the education of the caregivers/parents about what can be expected and what role they may or may not play in facilitating the IPSG. In this regard, the following areas will be covered:

- Caregiver education

- The recording environment

- Preparation of the laboratory prior to recording

Preceding the procedural portion of the Atlas, Chapter 2 presents an overview of some of the basics of signal acquisition and processing. Since IPSG depends on the acquisition and display of bioelectric signals, an understanding of some of the principles of electricity and signal processing is a prerequisite to conducting IPSG. Although the fundamentals have changed little, the technology for acquisition, storage and manipulation is changing rapidly like all computerized applications as we move further into the 21st century. The specifics of various recording systems are not described.

REFERENCES

1. Kahn A, Dan B, Groswasser J, *et al.* Normal sleep architecture in infants and children. *J Clin Neurophysiol* 1996;13:184–97

2. Anders T, Emde RL, Parmelee A, eds. *A Manual of Standardized Terminology, Techniques and Criteria for Scoring of States of Sleep and Wakefulness in Newborn Infants.* Los Angeles, CA: UCLA Brain Information Service/BRS Publications Office, 1971

3. American Thoracic Society. Standards and indications for cardiopulmonary sleep studies in children. *Am J Res Crit Care Med* 1996;53:866–78

4. Guilleminault C, Souquet M. Sleep states and related pathology. In Korobkin T, Guilleminault C, eds. *Advances in Perinatal Neurology.* New York: Spectrum Publications, 1979:225–47

5. Hoffman E, Havens B, Geidel S, *et al.* Long-term continuous monitoring of multiple physiological parameters in newborn and young infants. Procedural manual. *Acta Paediatr Scand Suppl* 1977;266:5–24

6. Hoppenbrouwers T. Polysomnography in newborns and young infants: sleep architecture. *J Clin Neurophysiol* 1992;9:32–47

7. Hoppenbrouwers T, Hodgman JE, Arakawa K, *et al.* Polysomnographic sleep and waking states are similar in subsequent siblings of SIDS and control infants during the first six months of life. *Sleep* 1989;12:265–76

8. Curzi-Dascalova L, Mirmiran M. *Manual of Methods for Recording and Analyzing Sleep-Wakefulness States in Pre-term and Full-term Infants.* Paris: Les Editions INSERM, 1996

9. Illingworth RS. Sleep problems in the first three years. *Br Med J* 1951;1:722–8

10. Dreyfus-Brisac C. Ontogenesis of sleep in early human prematurity from 21–27 weeks of conceptional age. *Dev Psychobiol* 1968;2:162–9

11. Dreyfus-Brisac C. Ontogenesis of brain bioelectrical activity and sleep organization in neonates and infants. In Falkner F, Tanner JM, eds. *Human Growth*, Vol. 3. New York: Plenum Publishing Corporation, 1979:157–82

12. Ellingson RJ, Peters JF. Development of EEG and daytime sleep patterns in normal full-term infants during the first 3 months of life: longitudinal

observations. *Electroencephalogr Clin Neurophysiol* 1980;49:112–24

13. Parmelee AH Jr, Wenner WH, Shulz HR. Infant sleep patterns: from birth to 16 weeks of age. *J Pediatr* 1964;65:576–82

14. Prechtl HFR, Beintema D. *The Neurological Examination of the Full-term Newborn Infant. Clinics in Developmental Medicine*, 12. London: Spastics Society and Heinemann, 1964

15. Aserinsky E, Kleitman N. Regularly occurring periods of eye motility and concomitant phenomena, during sleep. *Science* 1953;118:273–4

16. Aserinsky E, Kleitman N. A motility cycle in sleeping infants as manifested by ocular and gross body activity. *J Appl Physiol* 1955;8:8–11

17. Kleitman N. *Sleep and Wakefulness*. 2nd edn. Chicago: University of Chicago Press, 1963

18. Roffwarg HP, Muzio JN, Dement WC. Ontogenetic development of the human sleep–dream cycle. *Science* 1966;152:604–19

19. Parmelee AH, Stern E. Development of states in infants. In Clemente CD, Purpura DP, Mayer FE, eds. *Sleep and the Maturing Nervous System*. New York: Academic Press, 1972:200–28

20. Monod N, Pajot N. Le sommeil du nouveau-ne et du premature. I. Analyse des études polygraphiques (mouvements oculaires, respiration et EEG chez le nouveau-né à term). *Biol Neonat* 1967;11:216–47

21. Dittrichova J. Development of sleep in infancy. *J Appl Physiol* 1996;21:543–6

22. Parmelee AH, Wenner WH, Akiyama Y, *et al*. Sleep states in premature infants. *Dev Med Child Neurol* 1967;9:70–7

23. American Academy of Pediatrics. Clinical practice guidelines: diagnosis and management of childhood obstructive sleep apnea syndrome. *Pediatrics* 2002;109:704–12

24. American Academy of Pediatrics. Technical report: diagnosis and management of childhood obstructive sleep apnea syndrome. *Pediatrics* 2002;109:1–20

25. Consensus statement. National Institutes of Health Consensus Development Conference on Infantile Apnea and Home Monitoring, Sept 29 to Oct 1, 1986. *Pediatrics* 1987;79:292–9

26. Kelmanson IA. Circadian variations in the frequency of sudden infant death syndrome and of sudden death from life-threatening conditions in infants. *Chronobiologia* 1991;18:181–6

2

Basics of physiological signal acquisition and processing for infant polysomnography

In this Chapter, fundamental concepts are presented for obtaining and processing the signals used with the IPSG[1-6]. Engineering concepts are explained to an extent that they will be useful to the polysomnographer and PSG technologist. This Atlas does not, however, allow discussion at the level of detail necessary for a comprehensive understanding of these topics. Instead, concepts are included that are believed to be crucial for obtaining clinically optimal IPSGs.

BIOMEDICAL SIGNALS

Generally, *physiological signals* are considered to be 'time series', i.e. values of the physiological variable are given for every instant of time from a prescribed starting to a prescribed finishing time. Therefore, the physiological signal is said to be represented as a function of time.

Noise also can be represented as a time series. Noise can be defined as any other signal or random process that is not the desired signal. Random noise can be the result of fundamental properties of the materials and circuits that make up an electronic system or it can be interference by signals other than the one of interest. For example, noise can come from either man-made sources such as the 60-Hz power line waveform or random signals resulting from natural phenomena such as thunderstorms. In physiological signal acquisition, noise can also be other signals of physiological origin that are picked up along with the desired physiological signal.

In discussing a physiological signal, it is important to quantitatively relate its strength with respect to the noise in the channel. This is done using the *signal-to-noise ratio*. This is simply the ratio of the signal amplitude, energy or power to the noise amplitude, energy or power. Signal-to-noise ratio is usually presented using a logarithmic scale originally developed for the measurement of sound intensity. This scale, known as the *decibel scale*, makes it possible to describe a wide range of signal-to-noise ratios using a small range of numbers. For example, a signal-to-noise ratio of 20 dB corresponds to an actual amplitude ratio of 10 (the signal amplitude is 10 times greater than the noise amplitude). A signal-to-noise ratio of 40 dB corresponds to an actual amplitude ratio of 100. Although many polysomnographers are concerned about the sensitivity of their amplifiers, the real issue is the signal-to-noise ratio. For weak signals, a high signal-to-noise ratio means that it is possible to amplify the signal further to increase its amplitude, but the small noise amplitude will also be amplified keeping the signal-to-noise ratio constant. If the amplifier, on the other hand, introduces noise into the system, the overall signal-to-noise ratio for the physiological variable will decrease.

Sampled signals

Although physiological signals are continuous functions of time, i.e. there are no gaps in the signals, instantaneous changes in signal level, or microscopically sharp corners, it is often not practical to represent them as a continuous function. For example, a signal segment over a finite period of time would require an infinite time series to fully represent it. Because it is usually not practical to deal with such a representation of the signal, periodic samples of the signal are taken so as to have a finite series of numbers to represent it. Each number represents the signal's value at a specific point in time, and these signals are plotted by connecting the points. When a signal is digitized for computer analysis, a sample rate or sampling interval is determined and a time series is created representing the signal sampled at that rate. Figure 2.1a shows a continuous signal and a sampled signal in Figure 2.1b that represents the continuous signal. Although sampled signals only represent points uniformly distributed over time, often a sampled signal is made to look quasi-continuous by extending a horizontal line segment from one sample point over the interval until the next sample is taken. This is illustrated in Figure 2.1c. Note that when a continuous signal is sampled and reconstructed in this way it is no longer truly continuous according to the definition given above. If the sample rate is sufficiently high, however, the signal can be approximated as being continuous.

Signals must be sampled for analysis by computer, and there is a fundamental rule of signal analysis that must be followed when preparing a signal for computer analysis. This rule is that the sample rate must be at least twice the highest frequency component contained in that signal[6]. Thus, a rapidly changing signal such as the ECG must be sampled at a high rate to acquire all of the information in the signal, while a slower signal such as the breathing waveform can be sampled at a lower rate. For this reason an ECG signal is best sampled at a rate of 1000 Hz or higher to obtain all of its information, and a slower signal such as breathing movement can be sampled at a much lower rate of 50 Hz (Table 2.1). In some cases it is not practical to sample signals such as the ECG at optimally high rates, and so lower sampling rates such as 200 Hz are used. When this is done the ECG still appears in its familiar form, but some details are missing and it is not suitable for some types of analysis such as determining heart rate variability. The important message is that to reproduce a signal faithfully it must be sampled at a rate greater than some minimal value. This rule is known as the Nyquist criteria[6].

Time and frequency domains

Mathematicians who study signals have demonstrated that any continuous signal can be represented as a function of time or as the sum of a series of sinusoids of described amplitude, frequency and phase. A simple example of this is a square wave as illustrated in Figure 2.2. In the *time domain* (Figure 2.2a), the familiar square wave is plotted as a function of time. It can be shown that this same square wave could be represented as the sum of an infinite series of individual sinusoidal waves starting at the frequency of the square wave and having frequencies that are odd multiples of this fundamental frequency. Such a series is illustrated in Figure 2.2b. If we add the set of sinusoidal waves shown in Figure 2.2b, we get the signal shown in Figure 2.2c. This signal has the general shape of a square wave, but it is not the same as the square wave of Figure 2.2a. This is because we are only looking at a portion of the infinite series of sinusoidal waves. The more components of this infinite series that we include in the sum, the closer the result will look like the original square wave.

Table 2.1 Typical sampling rates for the infant polysomnogram

Signal	Minimum sampling rate (Hz)
Electrocardiogram (ECG)	200
ECG for heart rate variability	1000
Electroencephalogram (EEG)	100
Electromyogram (EMG)	
full signal	1000
envelope*	100
Electrooculogram (EOG)	10
Nasal/oral air flow	50
Nasal CO_2	50
Inductance plethysmography	50
Pulse oximetry	
saturation signal	10
pulse waveform	50
Motion	
mercury switch	5
accelerometer	50

* The envelope of the EMG is a plot of the EMG amplitude over time rather than the actual signal, so high-frequency information is removed and the signal can be sampled at a much lower rate

Instead of plotting individual sinusoidal waves of a specified amplitude and frequency, we can represent these signals graphically as shown in Figure 2.2c. In this case, a point is indicated on the graph to represent each sinusoidal component of the square wave (Figure 2.2d). The x-coordinate of the point is the frequency of the sine wave it represents, and the y-coordinate is that sinusoidal wave's amplitude. This plot represents the square wave in the *frequency domain*. In the case of the square wave which is a periodic signal only, sinusoidal waves of discrete frequencies that are odd multiples of the square wave fundamental frequency are present, but in the case of more general continuous biological signals, there are many more frequencies and amplitudes present. For this reason, biological signals can be described in terms of their frequency range. For example, the frequency domain representation of the infant ECG will have most of its energy in a range of frequencies from 0.1 to 150 Hz. These frequencies are the *frequency range* of a particular signal. This is an important consideration in processing signals, since the range of frequencies will determine the minimum sampling rate in the case of computerized signals and the minimum amplifier bandwidth to avoid signal distortion.

OBTAINING BIOMEDICAL SIGNALS: THE SENSOR

A biomedical instrumentation system such as a polygraph consists of three general components as illustrated in Figure 2.3. Each of the three blocks serves a particular function. The *sensor* is the interface between the physiological system being measured and the electronic instrumentation represented by the other two blocks of the system. As with any interface device one must be concerned with both sides of the interface: the interaction between the sensor and the physiological system and the interaction between the sensor and the remaining electronic components. Sensors convert the physiological variables being measured to an electrical signal that can then be processed by the signal processing electronics and stored or displayed at the instrument's output. Numerous different types of sensors are used to obtain the various channels of the IPSG. Table 2.2 lists the various signals, the sensor used to obtain these signals, the range of the variable being sensed, and the bandwidth of these signals. The following paragraphs will describe the different types of sensors in more detail.

Table 2.2 Signals, sensors and their bandwidths for the infant polysomnogram

Signal	Sensor	Signal range	Signal bandwith (Hz)
Electrocardiogram (ECG)	biopotential electrodes	0–1.5 mV	0.1–150
Heart rate	from electrocardiogram	0–250 bpm	0–5
Electroencephalogram (EEG)	biopotential electrodes	0–50 mV	0–50
Electromyogram (EMG)			
raw signal	biopotential electrodes	0–1 mV	0–1000
envelope	biopotential electrodes	0–1 mV	0–5
Eye movement	infrared source and detector	0–2 mV	0–10
	piezoelectric sensor	0–10 mV	0–10
Electrooculogram (EOG)	biopotential electrodes	0–100 mV	0–10
Nasal/oral airflow	CO_2 sensor	0–40 mmHg	0–5
	thermistor	0–2°C change	0–5
Inductance plethysmography	inductance plethysmograph	—	0–10
Transthoracic impedance	biopotential electrodes	< 0.5% of baseline	0–10
Breathing movement	piezoelectric sensor	0–10 mV	1–10
Breathing motion	liquid metal strain gauge	—	0–10
Motion detection	mercury switch	on–off	0–1
Motion detection	accelerometer	—	0–10

Bioelectrical potentials – biopotential electrodes

Electrical signals of biological origin are one of the most frequently measured biophysical variables for diagnostic and investigative purposes. Four of these signals are used in the IPSG. The ECG is used to determine cardiac rate and rhythm. The EMG is an electrical signal resulting from the contraction of skeletal or smooth muscle that can be used to determine when that muscle contracts and to get a qualitative sense of the strength of contraction. The EEG is a signal detected on the surface of the scalp that is produced by ensemble brain cell activity. The EOG is an electrical signal seen on the skin surface in the vicinity of the eyes that is produced by the electrical properties of each eye and can be used to detect eye movements.

All of these electrical signals appear in the body and on its surface. To be measured by electronic equipment, these signals must be changed from their biological form to a form that can be processed by electronic devices. The *biopotential electrode* makes the necessary transformation by changing signals in the body based upon ion distributions to signals in wires based upon the transport of electrons.

There are several different types of biopotential electrodes that can be used for different biomedical applications[2]. These can be classified into two general categories: polarizable and non-polarizable. Polarizable electrodes include those fabricated from noble metals such as platinum or gold, or other metals such as stainless steel. When these electrodes come in contact with an ionic electrical conductor such as biological tissue, the skin surface, or electrode gel and paste, a thin layer of electrical charge known as the double layer is established in the ionic medium in contact with the electrode. This double layer of charge is formed as a result of the chemical reactions between the electrode metal and the ionic conductor. Because this double layer is in the ionic medium (the skin or the body), electrode movement can disturb this double layer resulting in an electrical signal of non-biological origin, which can interfere with the signal being measured. This interfering signal is often referred to as a *motion artifact*[7].

Non-polarizing electrodes have special chemical surfaces to minimize the build-up of the electrical double layer. The most common non-polarizable (although not perfectly non-polarizable) electrode in biomedical applications is the *silver/silver chloride electrode*[1,8]. This electrode minimizes double-layer formation by having a silver chloride surface. This results in lower motion-induced artifact and noise for silver/silver chloride electrodes when compared to noble metal electrodes such as gold.

Both silver/silver chloride and gold electrodes are used in obtaining the IPSG. Miniature gold-plated electrodes can be used to sense the EEG and EOG. Although they may be subject to more noise and artifact than the silver/silver chloride electrode, their small size, robust structure and relatively low cost frequently make them the electrode of choice in these applications. Miniature silver/silver chloride electrodes are also available for these applications. They frequently give a better performance than the gold electrodes, but in many cases the improvement is only slight and does not warrant the additional costs. Electrodes for picking up the ECG are almost always the non-polarizable silver/silver chloride sensor. These electrodes are available from many sources, and disposable electrode structures including the electrode and an adhesive pad are inexpensive and used in most clinical monitoring applications.

There are many physical, chemical and electrical characteristics to describe biopotential electrodes. Of these, one that is important to understand when applying these electrodes with the IPSG is the concept of electrode *source impedance*. An electrical current in any medium other than a superconductor encounters interference that limits the amount of current that can flow for a particular driving force. In the case of a direct current (DC) this interference is known as electrical resistance. In the case of time-varying or alternating current (AC) this interference is referred to as impedance. As the impedance increases, it is more difficult for the current to pass through the medium, and for an electrical insulator where no current can pass, the impedance is infinite. Impedance and resistance are similar in that resistance is one component of the impedance, but there are additional factors in impedance not found in the DC case.

Biopotential electrodes (and most other electronic devices) have an associated impedance. In the case of electrodes, this impedance is often referred to as the source impedance. It is a measure of how well the electrode is connected to the biological host as well as how well the electrode itself is functioning. A high source impedance can indicate that an electrode is not well connected to the biological source of the signals it is measuring. This can lead to poor recordings of that signal due to increased noise and artifact or distortion of the signal due to the poor connection. In recording the IPSG it is important to verify that the electrode connections are good before the recording begins and to confirm this at the end of the recording. Many IPSG recording devices have built-in instrumentation to allow the PSG technician to measure the source impedance of each electrode to determine if it is functioning properly. Actual source impedances differ from one type of electrode to another, but a general rule for EEG and EOG electrodes is that their source impedances should be lower than $10\,000\,\Omega$. Often the source impedance for non-polarizable electrodes such as the silver/silver chloride electrode is lower than for the equivalent size gold electrodes.

Respiratory signals

Respiratory signals are used to characterize the respiratory pattern and respiratory rate, to identify respiratory events such as central or obstructive apneas and hypopneas, and to determine the adequacy of gas exchange. These signals are generally indirect measurements of the true parameters of interest in order to maintain the minimally invasive nature of the IPSG.

Nasal–oral airflow

Indirect measurement of nasal and oral airflow is usually accomplished by two methods in the IPSG: the measurement of carbon dioxide (CO_2) content in the exhaled air[9], and measuring temperature differences between inhaled and exhaled air[10]. Both techniques involve placing a sensing structure near the mouth and nose so that it contacts the air entering and leaving the airway. In the case of measuring CO_2 content in the breathing air (capnography), the best approach is to place a small catheter just inside one of the nares so that it will sample the gas entering and leaving the airway. This fine-bore tubing continuously withdraws a gas sample from the airway and transports it to the proximal end of the tube where a miniature CO_2-analyzing sensor is located. The gas sample is passed over this sensor, and a signal proportional to the CO_2 content of the gas currently in the sensor is

produced. It is important to recognize that the nasal catheter must only sample a small percentage of the breathing air so that it does not disrupt airway airflow. For this reason and for being able to place the catheter in an infant's nose, only fine-bore tubing should be used. It should also be recognized that an interval of time is required for the gas sampled in the infant's nose to be transported along the tube to the location of the sensor. To minimize this time, the tube should be as short as possible without interfering with the infant. Most sleep laboratories are able to keep delay times in the range of 1–2 s. The CO_2 sensor itself must be small so that it can be located outside the remainder of the instrumentation close to the infant. Most modern CO_2 analyzers that are used in the sleep laboratory measure the CO_2 content of the sampled gas using an infrared optical technique. This type of sensor responds very quickly to changes in CO_2 concentration and does not add any delay beyond that imposed by gas transport through the collection tube.

Very low mass temperature sensors can also be used to detect breathing air movement. The temperature of exhaled air will be higher than that of inhaled air, so a rapidly responding temperature sensor in the air stream as it enters and leaves the airway can be used to sense breathing. Miniature temperature sensors, known as *thermistors*, are usually used as the temperature sensors. These devices can be made to be very small and, therefore, have a very low mass so that they respond quickly to temperature changes. Thermistors are electrical devices in that they change their electrical resistance as the temperature changes. They are very sensitive and can have resistance changes as great as 5% per degree centigrade. Probes containing a thermistor, located under each nostril, are used for the nasal air temperature measurement. In some cases, there is a third probe that can be placed over the mouth so that oral breaths are detected as well. The output can display the nasal and oral information separately or reflect the sum of the three probes.

A disposable nasal/oral temperature sensor based upon thick-film microelectronic technology has also been developed for the direct measurement of infant and adult breathing (Eden Tec Corp, Eden Prairie, MN, USA). This device also changes its electrical resistance as the temperature of the air moving across its surface changes. By using a thick film, the sensor can have a large surface area for heat transfer while maintaining a low mass so that its thermal response will be rapid.

It is important to note that both the airway CO_2 sensor and the temperature sensor are not true flow sensors. In the former case, the CO_2 in the expired alveolar air is sensed, while in the latter case it is the temperature of the exhaled air that is detected. If each of these sensors were ideal and responded instantaneously, the breathing pattern that they detect would look like a rectangular wave rather than the expected almost sinusoidal breathing pattern as shown in Figure 2.4. The reason rectangular waves are not seen in practice is that neither sensing system is ideal. Even though the CO_2 sensor responds rapidly, there is mixing of gas at the interface between the alveolar gas and the adjacent gas in the airway dead space. This mixing not only occurs in the airway, but it can also occur to a lesser extent in the tube connecting the airway to the CO_2 sensor. Rounding of the corners of the temperature waveform is the result of the non-instantaneous response time of the temperature sensors. Even though the low mass causes them to respond rapidly, this response is not instantaneous as heat must be transferred from the gas that passes over them to the sensor itself. Since this response is not instantaneous, it often appears that breaths of increased tidal volume or extended duration appear to have higher amplitudes than shorter, smaller breaths. The larger, longer breaths produce this increase in amplitude because there is more time and more warm air volume to allow the temperature sensor to reach a higher temperature than is possible with the shorter, smaller breaths. It is important to understand this difference in thermally sensed breath amplitude and to recognize that if it is related to differences in tidal volume, the relationship is not a reliable one and one should be careful in interpreting amplitude differences in air temperature recordings. Thus, neither of these sensors can truly measure hypopnea, since they do not measure tidal volume. Nevertheless, some investigators have found that the nasal cannula and CO_2 instrumentation provide better indications of hypopnea than the temperature sensors[11].

Another important difference between the CO_2 and air temperature measurements is illustrated in Figure 2.4. Note that the idealized CO_2 signal begins later in time than the idealized air temperature signal. This is due to the fact that there is only an elevation in CO_2 in the alveolar gas that is exhaled while both the alveolar and dead space gas will have an elevated temperature. Since the dead space gas is exhaled before the alveolar gas, the temperature sensor will respond more quickly than the CO_2 sensor. Both will, however, indicate the same time for the end of exhalation.

Transthoracic impedance

One of the most common methods of monitoring infant breathing is the measurement of transthoracic electrical impedance[12]. As with biopotential electrodes, there is an electrical impedance associated with passing an AC current through the body. The higher this impedance is, the more difficult it is to pass the current through the body. The electrical impedance of the thorax varies by a small amount over time. The sources of this variation are changes due to the breathing and cardiac cycles. When the lungs are fully inflated, their electrical impedance, and hence that of the entire thorax, increases because air is not a conductor of electricity. Similarly, when the chambers of the heart are filled with blood, their impedance drops because blood is a relatively good conductor of electricity. Thus, if one measures the electrical impedance between two electrodes placed on the chest, a baseline impedance value is seen due to the impedance of the thoracic tissues and the impedances of the electrodes. This impedance is seen to increase by a small amount as the subject inhales air and to decrease when the air is exhaled. This variation in impedance as seen from the skin surface is generally quite small being only about 0.5% of the baseline impedance. Similarly, impedance variations are seen that correspond to the cardiac cycle. Generally, these impedance variations are even smaller than those due to respiration, and if transthoracic impedance is to be used to monitor breathing these variations in impedance as a result of the beating heart are considered to be artifact and should be minimized. It is usually not possible to eliminate the cardiogenic artifact completely but it can be minimized by careful choice of electrode positions.

Although the measurement of transthoracic electrical impedance is commonly used in infant breathing monitoring, it does have some limitations that the polysomnographer should be aware of. Transthoracic electrical impedance monitors are sensitive to all variations in impedance whether they come from the infant or not. As noted in the previous section, biopotential electrodes have an impedance associated with them. Much of this impedance is the result of the double layer of charge that forms on the electrode surface. As noted earlier, moving the electrode disturbs this double layer resulting in electrical potential artifact. In addition, this disruption of the double layer causes electrode impedance variations that will be added to the impedance of the biological tissue to which the electrodes are connected. Such motion-induced impedance variations are frequently larger in amplitude than those variations due to breathing, and so movement of the subject can produce artifacts in the transthoracic impedance signal that completely obliterate the breathing waveform.

A second limitation of the transthoracic electrical impedance signal is that it is often unable to detect obstructive apnea. Even though no air is transported through the airway during obstructive apnea, geometric changes in the lungs and chest wall can result in changes in the transthoracic impedance. These changes can produce a signal that looks the same as a normal breathing signal even though the lungs are not ventilated. It is, therefore, not possible to identify obstructive apnea from the transthoracic impedance signal. If transthoracic impedance measurements are combined with nasal/oral temperature measurements, apnea as indicated on the latter channel when breathing activity is indicated on the former can be a good demonstration of an obstructed breath. Thus, even though transthoracic impedance is not a good primary signal for observing breathing in the IPSG, when it is combined with the nasal/oral temperature recordings or the nasal CO_2 recordings, one is able to characterize breathing patterns more fully compared to when only a single sensor is used.

Liquid metal strain gauge

The mechanics of breathing involves changes in the cross-sectional area and circumference of the chest and abdomen. Changes in circumference can be measured using electrical devices that produce a signal related to changes in their length. These devices are known as strain gauges and are one of the primary sensors used to measure changes in length per unit length known as mechanical strain. Strain gauges, however, are usually designed for measuring

very small displacements and are themselves not very compliant. Thus, to place them on a relatively compliant structure such as the skin of an infant's chest or abdomen would result in the biological structure complying to the length of the strain gauge rather than the strain gauge following changes in biological length.

A more compliant strain gauge was invented for plethysmography of human limbs[13]. This device consists of a fine-gauge, thin-walled compliant rubber tubing (usually fabricated from silicone rubber with a diameter of from 1–2 mm) that is filled with mercury. Electrical contact is made to this mercury column at each end of the tube. Because the tube is compliant, it can be relatively easily stretched to almost twice its original length, and the internal column of mercury becomes longer and its cross-sectional area decreases as the tube is stretched. The longer, thinner column of mercury has a higher electrical resistance than the original unstretched column, and this electrical resistance can be measured between the electrical wires making contact with the mercury at each end of the tube. Thus, there will be an electrical resistance variation that will be proportional to the changes in length of the tube as the tube is stretched and released. This signal can be electronically processed and converted to a voltage that is proportional to the changes in length of the tube, and this voltage can be recorded on one channel of a polygraph. This device is known as a *liquid metal strain gauge*.

The liquid metal strain gauge can be used to measure infant breathing effort by stretching the gauge and attaching it to the chest and/or abdomen of an infant usually so that it is within a transverse plane. As the infant breathes, the strain gauge stretches and contracts with the breathing movements and offers little resistance to the infant's breathing effort. Strain gauges can be attached to a segment of the infant's thoracic or abdominal circumference, or they can be wrapped completely around the infant's chest or abdomen to give a signal proportional to changes in the entire circumference.

Liquid metal strain gauges have been shown to provide reliable breathing signals from infants in the research laboratory, and they have been used as breathing sensors in the sleep laboratory. They are inexpensive sensors, but they also have some limitations. Some polysomnographers may be concerned that these sensors contain elemental mercury, and there is a possibility that the silicone rubber tube may rupture during a study and expose the infant to this material. Such a scenario is not likely if the sleep laboratory technician is careful about how the sensor is applied and does not allow an individual sensor to be used for more than a few weeks so that old rubber that is more likely to rupture is not employed with patients/subjects. Nevertheless, the following warning should be heeded: liquid metal strain gauges contain elemental mercury, and their rubber tubing may rupture during use exposing patients/subjects and staff to this toxic material. Many hospitals will not allow sensors containing mercury to be used.

Another limitation of the liquid metal strain gauge is its susceptibility to noisy operation. Silicone rubber is easily penetrated by atmospheric gases, and oxygen in the air can result in the formation of oxides of mercury in the tube lumen. Since these oxides are not electrically conductive, they can interrupt the continuous column of mercury as the sensor is stretched, and this will result in a sharp increase in electrical resistance. Such increases appear as noise spikes on the recording of this signal. This problem can be reduced in a similar way to reducing the risk of rupture of the silicone rubber tube by avoiding the use of older sensors that have undergone multiple uses. Thus, it is important to replace sensors after several uses.

An alternative to the liquid metal strain gauge is the piezoelectric strain sensor[14]. A piezoelectric material is one that produces a small electrical signal when it undergoes a strain, and this can be used as a breathing sensor in much the same way as the liquid metal strain gauge without its attendant limitations. These strain gauges are generally not as compliant as those formed from rubber tubing, and so care must be taken in attaching them to infants to be sure that they are not adding significant mechanical resistance to infant breathing movements. These devices also have limitations in their low frequency sensitivity, so they may distort the breathing waveform when they are not electronically matched to the recording system.

The inductance plethysmograph

The liquid metal strain gauge measures changes in thoracic and/or abdominal circumference. Changes in thoracic and abdominal cross-sectional area can

also be measured as a way of determining breathing effort. When this is done, signals that are proportional to tidal volume can often be obtained since changes in cross-sectional area can be proportional to changes in lung volume.

An electrical property of a loop of wire known as its *inductance* changes in a way that is roughly proportional to the area subtended by the wire loop. The inductance of a wire loop can be measured using electronic circuits that produce a voltage that is proportional to the inductance signal. Thus, by placing wires around an infant's chest and abdomen in the form of two separate loops, it is possible to determine changes in the cross-sectional area by measuring changes in the inductance of these wires. This is what is done by the inductance plethysmograph. Since wire is stiff and not very compliant, it cannot be used directly to form the loops around the chest and abdomen. However, if it is formed in the shape of a sinusoidal wave, this can be attached to an elastic band such that, as the band is stretched, the sinusoids tend to be stretched out, and they return to their original shape when the band is relaxed.

The inductance plethysmograph measures changes in relative thoracic and abdominal volumes by measuring inductance changes in the wires of these elastic bands when one is placed around the chest and the other around the abdomen. By electronically processing these signals it is possible to obtain a signal related to the weighted sum of each individual signal that is proportional to tidal volume. In normal breathing this sum will be greater than zero, and the sum signal can be used to determine when a breath has been taken as well as its relative tidal volume. If the infant's airway is obstructed, there will be paradoxical movement in the chest and abdomen so that the signals from the chest band will be the inverse of those from the abdominal band. This is sometimes referred to as out-of-phase breathing. The weighted-sum signal in this case should be zero or near zero indicating the possible obstructed breath. Thus, this method of monitoring breathing allows the polysomnographer to identify possible obstructed breaths.

The inductance plethysmograph has been demonstrated to provide reliable signals for infant polysomnography[15]. Its advantage lies in the ability to recognize and differentiate possible obstructive apnea from central apnea. Its disadvantage lies in the complexity of the electronics needed to make this measurement and, therefore, the cost of the instrumentation. Disposable elastic band sensors are relatively inexpensive; therefore, the cost per individual subject monitored will be low if the cost of the capital equipment can be amortized over many subjects.

Measurement of hemoglobin oxygen saturation

The techniques described in the previous section for measuring breathing effort provide one way to assess the respiratory status of the infant. Another approach is to look at the outcome of the breathing process, that is, how well the cardiopulmonary apparatus is able to supply oxygen to peripheral tissues. The *pulse oximeter* is an instrument that has been developed for doing this non-invasively[16]. It functions by passing light at two different wavelengths (colors) through easily transilluminated portions of the body such as a finger, hand, toe or foot. A probe consisting of a near-infrared and a visible red light source is placed on one side of the structure being transilluminated, and a light detector sensitive to both wavelengths is placed on the opposite side so that it is illuminated through the tissue by the two light sources.

It is well known that fully oxygenated blood has a bright red color while blood with low oxygen content has a deep maroon color. The pulse oximeter determines oxygen content in the hemoglobin of the blood by looking at its color. The problem in doing this through tissue is that there are materials in the light path other than just blood, and these can interfere with the measurement. Two wavelengths of light are used in an effort to circumvent this problem. If one looks at the optical spectra of oxygenated and deoxygenated hemoglobin, it is found that there are big differences in the visible red portion of the spectrum but the actual characteristics cross one another in the near-infrared portion of the spectrum. By using two light sources and having one of them in the visible red portion of the spectrum and the other near the wavelength where the characteristics cross in the near-infrared portion of the spectrum, it is possible to normalize the changes in red coloration of the transilluminated tissue to the relative amount of blood in that tissue. Thus, one can separate out the effects of skin and deeper tissue pigmentation as well as blood volume on the measurement.

Another problem to be addressed is identification of the oxygen content of the arterial blood, when most of the blood in peripheral tissue is either capillary or venous blood. Thus, by measuring color variations in the blood in peripheral tissue, arterial, capillary and venous blood are measured all mixed together. The pulse oximeter is an instrument that uses electronic signal processing to separate the arterial component of this mixed-blood signal. The volume of blood in tissue changes over the cardiac cycle with maximum volume occurring during systole when fresh arterial blood enters the capillary network. The minimum in-tissue blood volume occurs at the end of diastole when some of the capillary blood has run off to the venous system. If one looks at the intensity of light passing through a transilluminated tissue, it is seen that there are small variations in this intensity that correspond to the cardiac cycle and are a result of changes in the optical properties of the blood as well as its volume in the tissue over the cardiac cycle. At systole the arterial blood has entered the capillaries, and the difference in optical properties of the tissue at this point from what they were at the end of diastole is due to this arterial blood. Thus, the pulse oximeter processes the small variations in light intensity seen by the photodetector as light at the two different wavelengths passes through the tissue.

It is important to understand the basic principle of this rather complicated analysis, because there can be other sources of pulsations in the light intensity seen by the photodetector that are not due to the arterial blood. These pulsations can lead to errors in determining the arterial blood hemoglobin oxygen saturation. The most common source of these variations is movement of the infant. Movement causes the path from the light sources to the light detector to change, and this results in small changes in the received signal. Often these changes are able to masquerade as arterial blood pulsations or they can be sufficiently strong to completely obliterate the actual pulsations due to the arterial blood. When this occurs it confuses the electronic signal-processing algorithm of the pulse oximeter, and causes an incorrect calculation of arterial blood hemoglobin oxygen saturation.

Movement of a limb with a pulse oximeter probe can create changes in the venous blood volume in that limb due to hydrostatic pressure changes. These volume changes can also result in pulsations of the light passing through the tissue, and the instrument cannot usually differentiate between these venous pulsations and arterial ones. In this case, since the hemoglobin oxygen saturation in venous blood is lower than that in arterial blood, these pulsations can lead to erroneously low measured arterial hemoglobin oxygen saturation.

Because of these situations, it is important to evaluate pulse oximeter readings critically to be certain that they are detecting the true arterial signal and not an artifact. The best way to do this is to look at the pulse signal produced by the light passing through the transilluminated tissue to determine if pulses are present and if they correspond to the cardiac cycle. It is also important that these pulses do not have wide amplitude variations that are usually associated with movement. If it is not possible to do this, then the polysomnographer should only accept pulse oximeter readings when there is no movement of the infant as indicated by other IPSG channels.

Pulse oximeters utilize electronic signal processing in an effort to reduce readings that are in error. The most common technique is to average the amplitudes of several detected pulses to minimize the effects of occasionally large or small pulses. This averaging can, however, reduce the response time of the instrument while it is reducing artifacts, and small transients in the actual signal might be minimized by this process. It is important for the polysomnographer to be aware if the pulse oximeter being used is averaging the signal as well as knowing over how long a time-window the pulses are being averaged. Ideally, pulse oximeters that do not average the signal should be used, but this often significantly increases the noise content of the signal.

Movement and activity sensors

Even though it is often obvious from a polysomnogram that the infant being studied is moving, it is helpful to have a direct indication of infant movement. This helps to identify the source of artifacts on the other channels of the polysomnogram, and it is a valuable signal in and of itself for determining and verifying sleep state. Movement sensors are found in various forms ranging from very simple switches to more complicated multi-axis accelerometers[17]. Examples

of these sensors are illustrated in Figure 2.5. A *mercury switch* consists of a glass capsule containing a pool of mercury with two electrical contacts passing through the glass wall at one end of the capsule. When the mercury is at that end of the capsule due to gravity, an electrical circuit is completed between the two electrical contacts (Figure 2.5a). If, however, the device is positioned so that the mercury moves to a different location in the capsule, electrical continuity between the two contacts is lost. Motion is detected by attaching a mercury switch such as this to a limb of an infant being studied with the capsule positioned to allow the mercury to complete the electrical circuit, when the infant is resting or sleeping quietly. Movement of this limb will relocate the mercury in the capsule interrupting the electrical circuit, even if only for a very short instant of time, and this can be recorded by an event recorder channel or a data channel of the polysomnograph.

The advantage of the mercury switch for measuring infant movement is that it is a simple device that is relatively inexpensive. Unlike the liquid metal strain gauge, mercury switches are robust and there is little likelihood of the capsule rupturing during a study exposing the infant to elemental mercury. The primary limitation of this device is that it will respond only to certain types of movement that will relocate the mercury in the capsule. It is also unable to indicate the relative level of activity of the particular movement. Either the switch responds to the movement or it does not.

More complicated activity-sensing switches have been developed that are based on the simple mercury switch principle of operation. An example of this kind of switch is illustrated in Figure 2.5b. In this case, the capsule becomes a circular cylinder with a series of electrical contacts evenly positioned around its periphery. A central electrode on one of the bases of the cylinder is always in contact with the mercury drop within the chamber. This device is attached to an infant's limb, and, as the infant moves, different contacts along the periphery of the sensor will encounter the mercury drop, and electrical continuity will be established between the central electrode and peripheral electrodes depending on the location of the mercury. Electrical contact between several different peripheral electrodes will be established and broken, with the particular electrodes involved being determined by the position of this sensor on the infant and the magnitude of the movement being measured.

Since this sensor is more complicated than the simple mercury switch, it is also more expensive and requires a more extensive electronic circuit to produce a signal for recording. This signal is better able to represent the movement than the signal from a single mercury switch, but it still does not truly quantitate the movement. Nevertheless, this device is quite popular as an infant activity sensor.

Miniature *accelerometers* are sensors that measure acceleration (Figure 2.5c). In recent years, very small accelerometers have been developed using silicone micromachining technology, and these are important components in automobile safety systems and other applications. These same devices can be used as motion sensors in the IPSG. Accelerometers sense movement of the infant. Accelerometers also pick up the acceleration due to gravity, and this signal can either be used to determine infant position or filtered out so that the remaining signals represent small accelerations due to infant movement. The simplest accelerometers (and the smallest) only measure acceleration in one direction, so it is important when using these sensors on infants that they are placed so that the most likely infant movements are in the direction of the accelerometer's sensitivity.

Accelerometers can be attached to infant limbs or more centrally depending on the type of movement one wishes to measure. Packaged accelerometers can be as small as infant biopotential electrodes and can be attached to the infant in a similar manner using an adhesive material. Miniature accelerometers should be placed in a robust package so that they are less susceptible to damage and can be used many times. Of the three types of sensors described, the accelerometer is most likely to detect infant movement and provide a quantitative measure of its intensity.

Eye movement

Eye movements are frequently monitored using the electrooculogram (EOG). In this case, small biopotential electrodes placed lateral to the eyes sense small electrical signals resulting from a small electric field produced by the eye. In some cases in infants this signal is very small and difficult to

measure and so alternative methods have been developed. One of these involves monitoring the reflection of a very low intensity infrared illumination of the eye, with the lid either open or closed[18]. When the eye is stationary the reflected light intensity remains constant, but when the eye is moving there is a time-varying component of the reflected light that is sensed by a photodetector. The infrared light source and photodetector can be housed in a silicone elastomer cap that is placed over one eye and secured by non-allergenic tape.

A second method involves sensing small movements of the tissue surrounding the eye using a very small piezoelectric sensor taped on the face near the eye[19]. The small movements of the tissue are converted to very small electrical signals by the piezoelectric material, and these signals will have a characteristic pattern when there is rapid eye movement.

Gastric acid reflux

The measurement of the acidity of the esophagus and the clearance of esophageal acid is an assessment that is sometimes used in IPSG. The measurement technique involves the use of a miniature *pH sensor* that can be placed in the esophagus. An external reference electrode such as a biopotential electrode on the skin surface may be necessary to complete the electrical circuit for this measurement. The pH sensor is similar to a biopotential electrode in that it produces a voltage that is related to pH (or acidity) of the medium that it contacts. There are many different types of pH sensors available to analytical chemists, but only two of these types have been used for esophageal pH measurement. The first is the antimony/antimony oxide electrode[20]. This usually takes the form of a small pellet of the metal antimony with an antimony oxide layer on its surface. This sensor is at the end of a flexible wire, and it can be passed into the esophagus of the infant through a nasal–gastric cannula. Older children and adults can advance this sensor into the esophagus by swallowing it with a drink of water. As gastric acid enters the esophagus, the pH in the region surrounding the sensor drops, and this causes the voltage measured between this electrode and a suitable reference electrode, for example, the skin electrode, to change.

Another type of sensor that is used for measuring reflux of gastric acid into the esophagus is a miniature *glass pH electrode*[21]. Larger versions of this sensor are routinely used in chemistry laboratories to determine the pH of a solution. Miniature sensors, 2–4 mm in diameter are available as combination electrodes; that is, they contain both the glass electrode and a reference electrode placed at the end of a flexible cable. This sensor can be advanced into the esophagus or swallowed just as the antimony/antimony oxide electrode, and it will produce an electrical voltage that is related to the pH of the medium in the vicinity of the sensor.

There are several differences between the glass electrode and the antimony/antimony oxide sensor. The former has a very high electrical source impedance, and this can lead to noisy recordings or interference from other electrical sources. Since this sensor is made of glass, it can also be fragile, and while it is unlikely that such a sensor will break while being used in the esophagus, normal handling in the laboratory may cause breakage of the glass. A final difference between the two types of sensors is related to cost. Miniature glass electrodes can be very expensive compared to the antimony/antimony oxide electrodes.

PROCESSING BIOMEDICAL SIGNALS

A medical instrumentation system must take the signal from a biomedical sensor and manipulate it into a form that can be useful for the measurement being made. The *processor* section of a general instrument (Figure 2.3) is the block of the instrumentation system that does this. One can describe the general activity of the processor block as electronic modification of a signal. There are several different functions that a processor block can carry out, but this discussion is limited to those processes that are directly related to polysomnography[6].

Amplification

As seen earlier in this Chapter, one of the ways of describing a signal is in terms of its amplitude as a function of time. Very often the amplitude of signals at the output of a sensor is too small to be useful. Amplification is a method of processing a signal to increase the amplitude by a factor greater than one and this factor is known as the *gain* of the amplifier. Amplifiers can increase signals to many thousand times their original amplitude to allow them to be

observed and/or recorded. If a biomedical signal in the frequency domain is considered, an amplifier should have the same gain for all frequency components of that signal. If this is not the case, the amplified signal will be distorted and will have a waveform different from that of the original signal. Figure 2.6 illustrates the process of amplification.

Amplifiers on polygraphs have gain controls to adjust the gain to the characteristics of a particular signal. These controls are often calibrated, not in terms of the gain factor but rather how large a signal at the input is needed to produce a specified deflection on a signal recorder or monitor screen at the output. For example, a typical gain setting would be 1 mV/cm on the output device. One might consider that the more gain an amplifier can provide the better it is for the signal. This is not true for two reasons. All amplifiers introduce a certain amount of noise into a signal as it is being processed, and this noise is often increased along with the signal. Thus, a very high gain amplifier will not only have the ability to increase the very weakest signals to the point where they can be observed, but it will also introduce a lot of noise on top of that signal, and this noise may in fact obliterate the signal itself. The signal and noise characteristics of an amplifier can be described in terms of its signal-to-noise ratio as noted previously. For example, an EEG signal that might have an amplitude of 25 μV could be amplified by an amplifier with a gain of 10 000 to produce an output voltage of 0.25 V. If this amplifier introduces the equivalent of 2.5 μV of noise to the signal at its input, there will be 0.025 V of noise on top of the signal. In this case, the signal-to-noise ratio will be 10. It is always good to have amplifiers with very high signal-to-noise ratios, for this indicates that the amplifier does not inject a large amount of noise into the signal.

The second problem with having the amplifier gain too high is that amplifiers cannot handle large voltage excursions at their output. For example, the ECG in Figure 2.7a has a maximum amplitude of 1.0 mV; if it is amplified with a gain of 1000, the output ECG will have an amplitude of 1 V. If the EEG amplifier of the previous example was used, which had a gain of 10 000, the output voltage amplitude would be 10 V. If this amplifier, however, had a maximum output voltage excursion of 5 V, it would not be able to reproduce the entire ECG faithfully. What would result is shown in Figure 2.7b where the peak of the ECG R-wave has been cut off due to the amplifier's inability to provide a signal at its output of greater than 5 V amplitude. This type of distortion is referred to as *saturation*, and it can be seen when the amplifier gain is too high for the signal being processed.

Offset

Sometimes a signal presented on a monitor screen or a chart recorder is not well centered on its recording channel. This can lead to saturation distortion as described in the previous section causing some of the signal to be cut off from the display or recording. The process of *offset* adds or subtracts a fixed voltage to a signal to move it up or down on the display or recording. Offset controls are often found on amplifiers and allow the operator to adjust the offset voltage continuously from a minimum to a maximum value. These controls can also be referred to as position or zero position controls.

Filtering

Although an amplifier processes a signal by multiplying all frequency components of that signal by a fixed gain factor, a *filter* is an electronic circuit that has a gain or attenuation factor that favors certain frequencies over other unfavored frequencies. Those frequencies that the filter favors are known as *pass frequencies*, while those that are not favored are known as *reject frequencies*. While amplifiers should always have a gain that is greater than one, filters can have output-to-input signal ratios that are less than unity for pass frequencies and are much less than unity for those frequencies that are rejected.

There are four common types of filters that may be used in polysomnography. The *high-pass filter* is a circuit that is designed to allow signal components at frequencies above a prescribed cut-off frequency to be passed while those below the cut-off frequency are rejected. A *low-pass filter* is just the opposite. Signal frequency components that are below the cut-off frequency are passed while those above the cut-off frequency are rejected. A *band-pass filter* passes a range of frequencies while rejecting those signal frequency components either above or below that range of frequencies. Band-pass filters are often described by their center frequency and their bandwidth, the frequency range from their low cut-off frequency to their high cut-off frequency. The final type of filter used in polysomnography is the *band reject* or *notch filter*. This filter rejects a range of frequencies but allows all other frequencies to pass. When the range of frequencies is narrow, this filter is referred to as a notch filter. Notch filters are sometimes used to reject interference from the power mains at either a frequency of 60 or 50 Hz. Of course, signal frequency components in the band reject range of the notch filter will also be eliminated, and this may cause the signal to be somewhat distorted.

Filtering is a strategy that can be used to improve the signal-to-noise ratio of an instrumentation system. If a source of noise covers a frequency range different from the signal being measured, a filter may be used to allow the signal being measured to pass while rejecting the frequencies of the other interference or noise. If the filter, however, affects frequencies in the frequency domain representation of a signal, that signal will be distorted. Thus, when noise has frequency components that overlap frequency components of a signal, one can reduce this noise by filtering, but this will also change the appearance of the signal.

Figure 2.8 illustrates how high-pass and low-pass filtering changes the appearance of an ECG. Trace a is the original infant ECG, while trace b shows this ECG processed with a low-pass filter having a high cut-off frequency of 25 Hz. Trace c shows the same ECG passed through a high-pass filter with a cut-off frequency of 1 Hz. Note that the high-pass filtered ECG has a distorted baseline and the T-wave has become biphasic. The S-wave has also developed an increased amplitude after passing through the filter. High-pass filtering of this type is sometimes used to remove baseline variations from an ECG and can reduce some types of motion-induced artifact. Although the ECG processed with this filter is distorted, it is still possible to observe the cardiac rhythm, so filtering of this type is often applied in long-term monitoring situations as a way to diminish motion artifacts.

The low-pass filter distorts the ECG by removing sharp corners. Note that the R-wave amplitude is lower in the filtered signal than it is in the original signal in Figure 2.8. Furthermore, the peak of the R-wave is rounded due to the filtering process. Once again, one is able to determine the cardiac rhythm after the ECG has been filtered in this way, but accurate determination of the location in time of the R-wave peak as it is used in heart rate variability analysis may be reduced as a result of this filtering.

ANALOG-TO-DIGITAL CONVERSION

As we shall see in subsequent chapters modern polygraphs involve computers and digital processing of the computer signals. The biological signals that we have discussed so far, however, are *analog* signals; that is, they are voltages that vary in time in proportion to the physiological quantity that they represent. To be able to process these analog signals on a digital computer, it is necessary to convert them into a *digital* format that consists of a number representing the value of the signal at predetermined, uniformly spaced intervals of time. The electronic circuit function that carries out this conversion is known as an analog-to-digital converter. This circuit samples the analog signal at a predetermined, uniform rate and generates a digital word representing the value of that signal at each sampling time. Thus, a digital signal is not a continuous signal in the true sense of the word in that it represents a finite number of samples. This is illustrated in Figure 2.1 where we see an analog signal and its sampled digital representation. It is obvious from this Figure that if there are changes in the analog signal that occur more rapidly than the sampling frequency, this information will be lost. Thus, it is important that the sampling frequency be high enough to represent the analog signal in an accurate way. A well-known theorem in electronic signal processing is the *sampling theorem*. This theorem shows that the sampling rate for a signal must be at least twice the highest frequency component of the analog signal (the Nyquist criteria) for the digital signal to represent its analog counterpart fully. In practice it is best to have the sampling rate at least five times the highest frequency component of the signal, since there are issues related to filtering and reproduction of the signal that are easier to handle when the signal is over-sampled in this way.

The sample rate of an analog signal then depends on the characteristics of the signal itself, and specifically its frequency spectrum, so that the highest frequency component of the signal can be determined. Table 2.1 gives some examples of typical sampling rates used in processing the various signals of the IPSG. It is important to note that these are typical sampling rates, and other rates may be used depending on the particular situation and type of analysis involved. Digital signals need to be stored on some sort of computer memory such as a floppy disk, hard disk, digital audio tape (DAT), or writeable CD-ROM or DVD-ROM. The higher the sampling rate, the more memory space is required for storing a given signal, so even though the highest fidelity of reproduction is obtained with higher sampling rates, practical issues of storing the data, as well as processing them on a computer, suggest that sample rates should not be artificially higher than necessary.

The range and resolution of a digital signal is another factor that affects the size memory required to store that signal. Most analog-to-digital converters used for biomedical signal acquisition have a resolution of 8, 12 or 16 bits. This indicates the number of divisions that the range of amplitudes of the signal can be divided into for purposes of digitization. For example, an 8-bit analog-to-digital converter can represent a signal with $2^8 = 256$ individual levels. Thus, a signal that has a range of 0–1 V would have a resolution in amplitude of $1/256 = 0.0039$ V. Variations of less than that value would not be seen in the signal. An analog-to-digital converter that has 12 bits has 4096 different levels or a resolution over a 1 V range of 0.000244 V; and a 16-bit analog-to-digital converter has 65 536 individual levels yielding a 1 V range resolution of 0.0000153 V. Thus, the higher the number of bits converted by an analog-to-digital converter, the better the resolution. More bits, however, also means that the digital words storing the information are longer and more memory is required. Roughly twice the memory is required to store one sample from a 16-bit analog-to-digital converter than required for an 8-bit analog-to-digital converter. Although most biomedical signals can be adequately reproduced using an 8-bit analog-to-digital converter, this assumes that the signals can be confined to a relatively narrow range. If the signals suffer from a drifting baseline, the signal itself may only require a 1 V range at the output of the amplifier, but due to the baseline drift, that 1 V may appear anywhere from -5 V to +5 V, and one needs a wider range for the analog-to-digital converter to avoid saturation errors due to the limits of the range.

SUMMARY

In this Chapter, some of the technical issues in terms of obtaining and processing biomedical signals used in the IPSG have been examined. It must be stressed that the discussion here is not a complete one but rather covers what are considered to be essentials for someone trying to obtain the IPSG. Engineering issues regarding sensing and signal processing are major subjects in the field of biomedical engineering and involve many technical issues not covered in this Chapter. Instead, the focus has been on issues related to description of signals, obtaining the signals used in the IPSG, and those steps of signal processing that are commonly applied with this diagnostic procedure.

REFERENCES

1. Webster JG, ed. *Medical Instrumentation, Application and Design*. 3rd edn. New York: John Wiley, 1998

2. Geddes LA. *Electrodes and the Measurement of Bioelectric Events*. New York: John Wiley, 1972

3. Richard S, Cobbold C. *Transducers for Biomedical Measurements: Principles and Applications*. New York: John Wiley, 1974

4. *Infantile Apnea and Home Monitoring, Report of a Consensus Development Conference*. NIH Publication No. 87-2905. Bethesda, MD:National Institutes of Health, 1986

5. Sackner JD, Nixon AJ, Davis B, *et al.* Noninvasive measurement of ventilation during exercise using a respiratory inductive plethysmograph. *Am Rev Resp Dis* 1980;122:867–71

6. Rangayyan RM. *Biomedical Signal Analysis, A Case-Study Approach*. New York: IEEE Press, 2002

7. Webster JG. Reducing motion artifacts and interference in biopotential recording. *IEEE Trans Biomed Eng* 1984;31:823–6

8. Janz GJ, Ives DJG. Silver-silver chloride electrodes. *Ann NY Acad Sci* 1968;148:210–21

9. Hagerty JJ, Kleinman ME, Zurakowski D, *et al.* Accuracy of a new low-flow sidestream capnography technology in newborns: a pilot study. *J Perinatol* 2002;22:219–25

10. Rigatto H, Brady JP. A new nose piece for measuring ventilation in pre-term infants. *J Appl Physiol* 1972;32:423–4

11. Trang H, Leske V, Gaultier C. Use of nasal cannula for detecting sleep apneas and hypopneas in infants and children. *Am J Resp Crit Care Med* 2002;166:464–8

12. Olsson T, Daily W, Victorin L. Transthoracic impedance: theoretical considerations and technical approach. *Acta Paediatr Scand Suppl* 1970;207:1–27

13. Whitney RJ. The measurement of volume changes in human limbs. *J Physiol (London)* 1953;121:127

14. Siivola J, Heikki LA. Non-invasive piezoelectric transducer for recording of respiration at the level of diaphragm. *Electroencephalogr Clin Neurophysiol* 1998;106:552–3

15. Brooks LJ, DiFiore JM, Martin RJ. Assessment of tidal volume over time in pre-term infants using respiratory inductance plethysmography. *Pediatr Pulmonol* 1997;23:429–33

16. Bowes WA, Corke BC, Hulka J. Pulse oximetry: a review of the theory, accuracy, and clinical applications. *Obstet Gynecol* 1989;74:541–6

17. Parker G, Gladstone G, Hadzi-Pavlovic D. Measuring psychomotor agitation by use of an actimeter: a pilot study. *J Affect Disord* 2002;72:91–4

18. Harper RM, Hoppenbrouwers T, Ross SA. A new technique for long-term recording of eye movements in infants. *Electroencephalogr Clin Neurophysiol* 1976;40:109–12

19. Pajot N, Vicente G, Dreyfus-Brisac C. Techniques d'enregistrement des mouvements oculaires chez le nouveau-né: comparaison des méthodes. *J Electrophysiol Technol* 1976;2:29–38

20. Jones RD, Neuman MR, Sanders G, Cross FT. Miniature antimony pH electrodes for measuring gastro-esophageal reflux. *Ann Thoracic Surg* 1983;33:491–5

21. Vandenplas Y, Goyvaerts H, Helven R, Sacre L. Gastroesophageal reflux, as measured by 24-hour pH monitoring, in 509 healthy infants screened for risk of sudden infant death syndrome. *Pediatrics* 1991;88:834–40

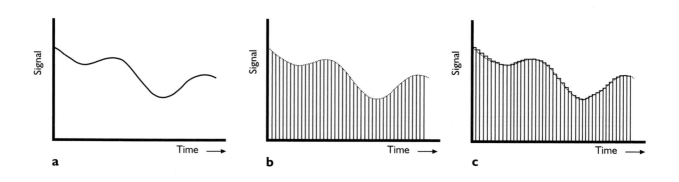

Figure 2.1 Example of a continuous signal and a sampled version of that signal. a, The continuous signal; b, the sampled version of the signal; c, a reconstructed version of the original signal from the sampled signal

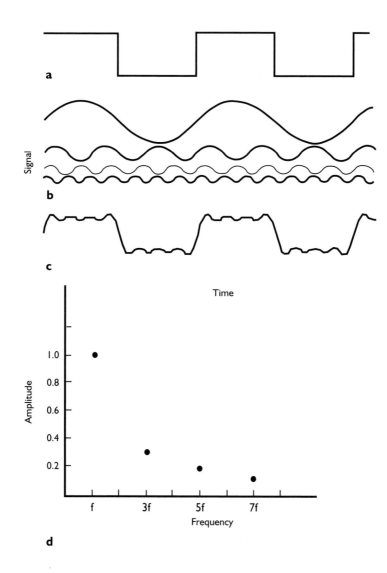

Figure 2.2 A square wave signal represented in the time and frequency domains. a, The original square wave in the time domain; b, the first four frequency components of the square wave and the sum signal for these four frequency components; c, the spectrum representing the square wave in the frequency domain; d, representation of the square wave in the frequency domain

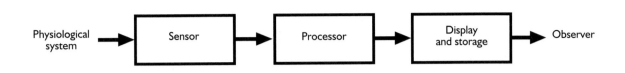

Figure 2.3 Block diagram of a general biomedical instrument

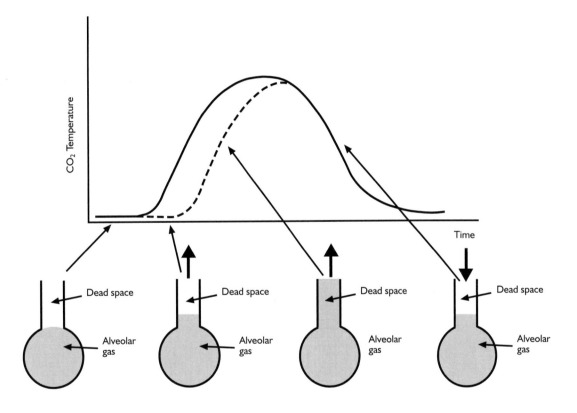

Figure 2.4 An example of an idealized CO_2, nasal airway temperature, airflow and volume curves obtained from an infant

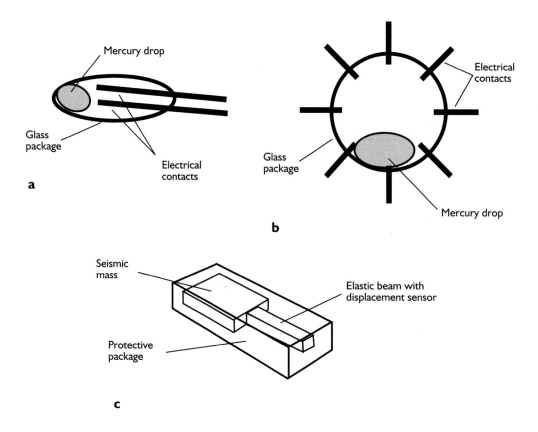

Figure 2.5 Sensors for detecting infant movement. a, A mercury switch; b, a multiple contact mercury switch; c, an accelerometer

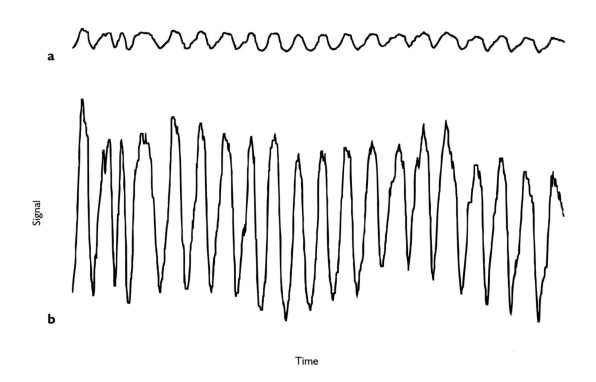

Time

Figure 2.6 Example of amplification of a biomedical signal. a, The original signal; b, the amplified signal

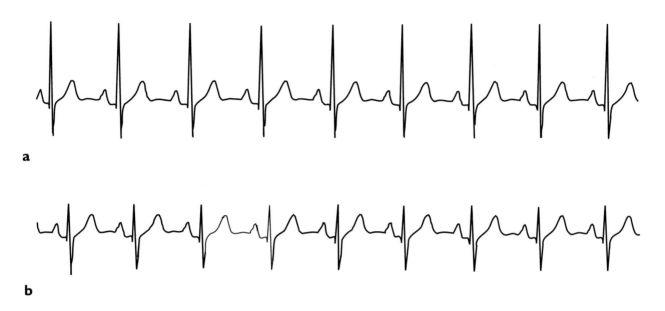

Figure 2.7 Saturation distortion in an electrocardiogram signal. a, The original electrocardiogram signal; b, the same signal with saturation distortion. Reprinted from reference 1, with permission

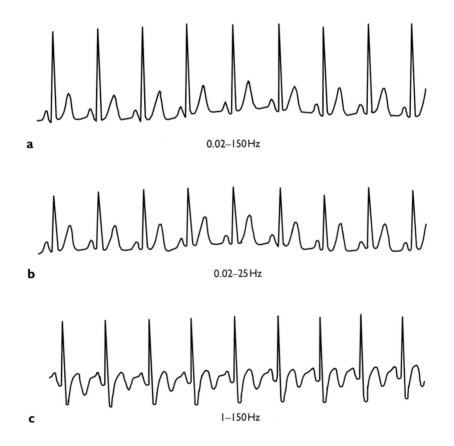

Figure 2.8 Frequency distortion of the electrocardiogram. a, The undistorted electrocardiogram; b, the electrocardiogram when passed through a low-pass filter with a cut-off frequency of 25 Hz; c, the electrocardiogram when passed through a high-pass filter with 1 Hz cut-off frequency. Reprinted from reference 1, with permission

3

Infant polysomnography recording procedures

With an appreciation and understanding of the fundamentals and purposes of the IPSG, the appropriate equipment and staffing can be assembled. This Chapter focuses on methods and considerations related to preparing for and conducting an IPSG. Good preparation and well-trained IPSG technicians are essential to achieving optimal recordings in infants. The expertise and infant handling skills of the technical staff are critical to infant and caregiver comfort levels and signal quality. The following sections provide detailed descriptions, directions and examples of pre-, during and post-recording procedures.

INPATIENT VS. OUTPATIENT IPSG

Sleep PSG laboratories may see infants as inpatients and/or outpatients. Most of the information in this Atlas avoids a distinction between these two settings. Each laboratory will have its own protocols for dealing with inpatient and outpatient studies. For those instances where infants are coming to the laboratory from home, and particularly where the parents will be staying overnight during the IPSG, caregiver preparation and education are crucial to obtaining an optimal study. An example of caregiver instructions is provided in detail in Appendix A.

DURATION OF MONITORING

As noted earlier, IPSGs can be as short or long as the purpose demands; that is, as short as a between-feeding nap or as long as overnight, possibly longer. The procedures described here can apply to any length of monitoring but were developed for the

all-night IPSG. Feedings, diaper changes and consoling must be anticipated especially in longer recording periods.

STAFFING

Infants should be under the *continuous* observation of trained personnel in sufficient numbers to observe the baby and to annotate the study properly. Two staff technicians are optimal, particularly during infant set-up. A single technician may suffice during monitoring if a parent is available to assist with routine baby care and there is ready access to emergency personnel.

RECORDING ENVIRONMENT

The laboratory should consist of two adjacent rooms, one for the sleeping infant and one for the equipment. The parent or caregiver may be instructed not to interfere with the infant during the study, but may sleep in a bed or reclining chair nearby. During the IPSG, the infant sleeping room should be under continuous surveillance through an audio-video monitoring system.

Staff must have easy access from the equipment room to the infant sleep room in case of emergency. Current certification in basic life support is a requirement for all IPSG personnel. There should be resuscitation equipment and an emergency cart as well as a system for alerting support personnel. An emergency plan should be developed and practiced. A sink, scale and other routinely used equipment should be handy. Carpeting is desirable so that arousals from noise are minimized; antistatic treatment should be considered. Overhead fluorescent lights should not be used during recording periods as they can introduce electrical noise into the recordings. Room temperature control is desirable for patient comfort. The infant sleep room is used for infant preparation. Infants must sleep in a crib or on a raised bed with sides that can be easily lowered. A summary of infant sleep laboratory requirements is provided in Table 3.1.

PREPARATION OF THE LABORATORY PRIOR TO THE INFANT'S ARRIVAL

Set-up of the sleep room

All materials and sensors required for the study should be available and determined to be in good working order. Do not wait for the evening to make sure all supplies are on hand and that equipment is functioning correctly.

Sensors such as the EEG, ECG and EMG should be checked for poor impedance levels (> 20 Ω) using an ohmmeter. Broken electrodes will need to be replaced.

Equipment set-up

The functioning of all recording and data acquisition devices should be checked regularly and during the day of the IPSG so that repairs and replacements can be obtained before the infant is scheduled to arrive. Preparation of the equipment will vary between laboratories, but there are some steps that will probably be useful in all settings.

Recording montage selection

The Current Procedural Terminology[1] guidelines for polysomnography include: 1–4 lead EEG, EOG and submental EMG. Examples of other parameters that can be added are additional EEG leads, ECG, airflow, ventilation and respiratory effort measures, gas exchange by oximetry, transcutaneous or end-tidal CO_2 monitoring, extremity muscle activity, motor-activity movement, gastroesophageal reflux, snoring and body position. The selected data acquisition

Table 3.1 Infant sleep laboratory requirements

Lighting	*Infant sleep room*
1. Preparation stage – standard overhead lighting	1. Video camera
2. Monitoring stage – 40 W adjustable lamp or infrared or black light	2. CO_2 monitor
Temperature	*Equipment monitoring room*
1. Ambient 23°C (approximately, depending on age of infant)	1. Monitoring system
	2. Video monitor/recorder
	3. Telephone
Bed	
1. Infant crib or hospital bed	
Infant supplies	*Associated equipment*
1. Diapers	1. Sink
2. Shirts	2. Scale
3. Blankets	3. O_2
4. Pacifiers	4. Suction
5. Suction bulb	
6. Formula/breast milk	*Emergency cart*
7. Sleeper	

Table 3.2 Infant–pediatric recording montage

Electroencephalogram (EEG) C3–A2

C4–A1

O1–A2

O2–A1

Electromyogram (EMG submental)

Electrocardiogram (ECG)

Respiratory effort

rib cage

abdomen

sum

End-tidal CO_2

waveform

numerical values

Nasal airflow

Oral airflow

Pulse oximetry

pulse waveform or perfusion index

SaO_2 percentages

Actimeter

Eye movement

left electrooculogram (LEOG)

right electrooculogram (REOG)

montage will depend on the purpose of the IPSG and the number of recording channels available. One example of a montage that includes the basic IPSG parameters is given in Table 3.2. Recording arrangements may vary as described in a recent summary in the American Thoracic Society *Standards and Indications for Cardiopulmonary Sleep Studies in Children*[2]. Electrode placements and definitions are described later in this Chapter. A summary of recording parameters can be found in recent reports from the American Academy of Pediatrics[3,4].

Calibration

Whether a paper recorder or computer-assisted data acquisition system is used, a set-up protocol is necessary to determine that all the amplifiers are functioning correctly. Calibration signals are typically set at 50 μV/7 mm or 10 mm. A series of these signals should be examined to determine that all AC amplifiers produce the correct amplitude and

pattern. The pattern or shape will vary depending on the filter settings. For the initial calibration all AC channels should be on the same settings to produce identical calibration waveforms (Figure 3.1a). Figure 3.1b shows a 30-s series of 100 μV calibration signals in the EEG, EOG and EMG channels that reflect the different waveforms produced by the different filter settings. These calibration patterns should be viewed as a double-check that filter settings are correct. Other calibrations usually must wait until the electrodes are applied and the signals can be recorded from all devices. Typically, written documentation is employed to verify that all the set-up tasks have been carried out and by whom. If problems are identified, attempted remedies and final solutions should be described. A sample of a checklist that can be used for this purpose is in Appendix B.

Electrode selection

Although electrodes and sensors suitable for infants are similar to those used in older children and adults, some consideration should be given to their size and methods of application to fragile infants. An array similar to that used in the CHIME study is listed in Table 3.3.

ELECTRODE APPLICATION

The electrode application process is critical to obtaining an optimal recording and equally important to reducing distress in the infant and, possibly, for the caregivers as well. Along with the specifics of applying the sensors to the body, the order of application can affect the outcome of an infant study. Infants are extremely sensitive to touching their heads and to placement of electrodes on the face. Therefore, it can be prudent to leave these sensors until last, or applying them during a feeding. As a last resort you can wait until the infant is asleep, but this may awaken the baby. A good feeding and burping can smooth the way as can the use of pacifiers, toys, and holding by parents or staff. The order in which sensors are applied is part of the sensitivity to the infant's response to handling. Table 3.4 shows one order of application as used by CHIME. Below, detailed descriptions of methods for applying each type of sensor are given.

ECG

Ensure that the baby's skin is dry and free of powder, oil or perspiration to provide good contact between the sensors and the skin. Two or three ECG electrodes will be applied (Figure 3.2a), using modified Lead 1 or Lead 2 placements (Figure 3.2b). The three electrodes permit changing from Lead 1 to Lead 2 if necessary without disturbing the infant. The two alternative placements graphically shown in Figure 3.2b may be required to obtain an optimal signal. In addition, the negative (-) and positive (+) electrodes reflect the polarity of the recorded heartbeat.

Respiratory effort

Inductance plethysmography or piezocrystal bands must be selected in the appropriate sizes for the baby. Place the top band around the ribcage at the level of the nipples (slightly above so as not to irritate the nipple) and the bottom band around the abdomen at the level of the umbilicus (Figure 3.3). It can be helpful to tape the bands in place to avoid their slipping out of position.

Oximeter sensor

Most neonatal/infant-sized oximeter sensors are a flexible semi-disposable or disposable type meant to be applied to the foot or hand (Figure 3.4). The sensor light source can be placed on the top of the foot (hand) taking care that the detector on the other side is directly *opposite* the light source. Use the opaque tape that comes with the sensor to fasten the sensor to the skin. Stretch-tape or a velcro-fastening band can be wrapped around the foot to secure it further and help eliminate the detection of ambient light. Care must be taken that any fasteners do not produce heat build-up. Changing the sensor position may be necessary during the recording period.

Position sensor

Application will vary according to the type of sensor. Apply according to the directions that accompany the sensor. Test to make sure that the appropriate tracing occurs when the infant is in the supine position. The site used by CHIME was the back of the diaper, affixed by tape (Figure 3.5).

Table 3.3   Typical electrode types for infant polysomnography

Electroencephalogram (EEG)	gold cup electrodes to be affixed to the scalp with paste
Electrooculogram (EOG)	miniature Ag/AgCl biopotential electrodes affixed with adhesive collars or gold cup electrodes
Submental electromyogram (EMG)	miniature Ag/AgCl biopotential electrodes affixed with adhesive collars or gold cup electrodes
Electrocardiogram (ECG)	pre-gelled ECG pad, hydrogel electrodes in infant and pediatric sizes, or Ag/AgCl biopotential electrodes
Airflow	nasal or nasal/oral airflow sensors and/or CO_2 sampling devices (tubing)
Respiratory effort	rib cage and abdominal bands; these can be inductance plethysmography bands, piezocrystal bands or equivalent
Position sensor	small size special purpose device
Motion sensor	accelerometer device in small, infant size or EMG-type leads on the legs/arms
Oxygen saturation	a neonatal/infant-size flexible sensor that can be taped to the foot

Ag/AgCl, silver/silver chloride; CO_2, end-tidal CO_2

Table 3.4 Suggested order for application of sensors

Body

Electrocardiogram

Respiratory bands

Oximeter sensor

Position/movement sensor

Head

Electroencephalogram

Electromyogram

Head wrap (such as cling bandage)

Face

Electrooculogram

CO_2 cannula

Neonatal/infant nasal/oral thermistor

Actimeter/movement sensor

Prior to placement on the baby, with the actimeter connected to the recorder, shake it gently to establish that it is operational. Deflections should appear on the recorder screen or paper if it is working. If not, use an alternate and repeat the test. Figure 3.6 is an example of an actimeter-activated body movement recording. Place the actimeter on the baby according to its directions with a consideration for infant comfort. Actimeter placement on the foot is shown in Figure 3.7. If leg leads are applied, they should be placed over the anterior tibialis muscle on each leg. If two recording channels are available, two leads can be placed on each leg from 1.3 to 2.5 cm apart. If only one channel is available, one electrode can be placed on each leg. Prepare the sites in the same manner as the submental EMG. To verify that the placement is adequate, the feet should be gently flexed to produce a phasic EMG burst similar to the submental EMG bursts in Figure 3.6 (underlined).

Submental EMG

Three electrodes of the type noted for EMG in Table 3.3 will be applied to sites on the chin: at the tip of the chin, on the right digastric muscle and on the left digastric muscle (Figure 3.8). Prepare the sites by briskly rubbing with alcohol on a gauze pad followed by rubbing with an abrasive cream/gel on a cotton-tipped applicator. Wipe off excessive cream/gel. Combinations of two of the three electrodes will be selected to obtain the best EMG signal. Priorities for insuring a good-quality signal can be established for each electrode combination; for example, first, tip of the chin and the right digastric, second, tip of the chin and left digastric, third, left and right digastric muscles.

EOG

The left EOG (LEOG) is placed 0.5 cm above and 0.5 cm away from the outer canthus of the left eye; the right EOG (REOG) is placed 0.5 cm down and 0.5 cm away from the outer canthus of the right eye (Figure 3.9a). Prepare the sites by briskly rubbing with alcohol on a gauze pad or with an abrasive cream/gel on a cotton-tipped applicator. Wipe off excess cream/gel. If using miniature biopotential electrodes, apply the adhesive collars and fill the well with electrode cream/gel. Ensure there are no air bubbles in the cream. Fill the well so that the cream will not ooze out under the adhesive collar when the electrode is pressed onto the skin. Remove the covering on the adhesive collar and press the electrode firmly onto the prepared site (Figure 3.9a). As noted, gold cup electrodes also can be used. Hydrogel electrodes are another alternative. Particular attention must be paid to protecting the eyes from liquids and pastes. Wires should be directed away from the face and into a 'pony tail' of all face/scalp lead wires. When additional eye-movement specificity is desired, two EOG channels can be recorded from both vertical and horizontal placements (see the diagram in Figure 3.9b). Two EOG channels also can be recorded from referencing both the LEOG and REOG placements in Figure 3.9a to A1 (M1).

EEG

EEG electrodes should be applied according to the International 10–20 measurement system[5]. The minimum array for IPSG would be the central sites C3 and C4 plus one or more reference sites such as A1 and/or A2. The A1 and A2 reference electrodes can be placed over the bony mastoid processes. When the mastoid is used the sites may be labeled as M1 and M2 (Figure 3.10). A ground electrode is always applied; one common site is the middle of the forehead (FPz) or closer to the hairline. Occipital leads, such as O1 and O2, are often added to the montage to document alpha frequencies and as alternatives if signals from the central leads are lost. A diagram of these sites is shown in Figure 3.10. A short-cut system for locating the central and occipital sites only is given in Appendix C. Prepare the sites by briskly rubbing with alcohol on a gauze pad and then with an abrasive cream/gel on a cotton-tipped applicator. Fill the gold cups with electrode paste and press onto the prepared site, direct the electrode wires to the back of the head. Cover the gold cup with a cotton ball or a small gauze square and tape as needed to secure the placement. After all impedances are checked, the entire head should be wrapped with cling bandage (Figure 3.11), so that the EMG and EOG electrodes are included for additional security. Impedances for all electrodes should be documented on a paper recording, on a checklist as in Appendix B or, if applicable, typed into the data acquisition computer comments.

Airflow

There are a variety of thermistors/thermocouples made specifically in infant sizes, most of which are positioned in front of the nares and mouth and secured by an adhesive backing or non-allergenic tape. Some IPSGs will use only one airflow sensor type, i.e. either a thermistor or thermocouple, or a CO_2 cannula. It is possible, however, to use both at the same time. Prior to placement, the staff can dip the thermistor or thermocouple sensor in and out of warm water to ensure that responses to cold/warm temperature changes are reflected on the recording. Be sure to dry the sensor after this test. The active sensor tips should be in front of but not touching the skin or inside of the nares (Figure 3.12).

If end-tidal CO_2 is part of the montage, the CO_2 cannula or tubing should be applied as the directions specify, inserted just slightly into the nare so that expired air can be sampled (Figure 3.13). Adequacy of the waveform can be observed on the capnograph.

OTHER INFANT SET-UP CONSIDERATIONS

In order to facilitate electrode/sensor placements, infant clothing is an important factor. Loose sleepers, like sacques, are useful in very small infants. Sleepers that snap down the front also help to provide easy exit and access to the electrodes and

sensors. In order to protect the electrode attachments, elbow covers ('No-No's') can be used so that the infant cannot bend his/her arms to reach the wires. The elbow covers do not otherwise affect infant movement. Infant-style velcro-fastening elbow covers make this procedure more palatable to caregivers. Supine or side-propped positioning is strongly advised to avoid interference with the sensors on the face.

In addition to testing signal quality as electrodes are applied, final checks as described in the 'Testing signal quality' section must be made prior to starting the officially defined sleep analysis recording period. This period is often defined by 'Lights out' to 'Lights on' or 'Begin study' to 'End study'. Every attempt should be made to achieve good electrode application the first time as most infants have a low threshold for repeated attempts to fix poor application.

If not already done, the next step is to interface the electrodes with the recording equipment. Most systems have specialized jack boxes or input devices for this purpose. Placing the electrode leads and ancillary equipment connections into the correct inputs is mandatory and should be carefully checked before any recording is started. The input connection arrangements and derivations will be determined by each laboratory.

TESTING SIGNAL QUALITY

Data acquisition should begin at this time, if not earlier, so that the signal quality testing can be recorded for later reference. Although infants cannot be asked to perform the maneuvers requested of older children and adults, signal quality can be assessed by observing spontaneously occurring behaviors. Some of the techniques used in the CHIME study are described below.

Eye movements

When the infant is awake, there should be a good quality EOG signal with the left and right EOG of opposite polarity to allow easy identification of eye movements. If the eye movements are recorded but are of the same polarity, check the position of the electrodes and the input device connections. Examples of opposite polarity and same polarity EOGs are in Figure 3.14a and b, respectively.

EMG

A good quality EMG signal will increase, that is, have phasic bursts of muscle activity, during crying and sucking (Figure 3.15). Adjust the gain, check electrode position, and/or plug in (or select) a different pair of EMG electrodes until a good-quality signal is obtained. If an ECG artifact is present in the EMG channel, choose a different combination of EMG electrodes. If active rapid eye movements (REMs) are observed during sleep prior to the start of the study, that is, during probable active sleep, adjust the gain on the EMG so minimal tonic activity will be recorded. The signal should not be totally removed since some muscle activity will then be lost.

Respiratory effort

Observe the baby's chest wall movement to determine that synchronous breathing, that is, inspiration and expiration are shown as the rib cage and abdomen deflecting in the same direction (Figure 3.16a). If the rib cage and abdomen appear to be out-of-phase, that is, inspiratory deflections in rib cage and abdomen move in opposite directions, look at the infant to verify that these signals are associated with paradoxical rib cage and abdomen movements (Figure 3.16b).

ECG

In the ECG the normal PQRST complex can be observed from the lead placements commonly used during IPSG (Figure 3.2b). A stylized example of the PQRST complex and an example from an IPSG are shown in Figures 3.17a and b, respectively. In the IPSG the R-waves should be 'up' and of sufficient amplitude for visualization of all the most prominent complex components. Optimal and poor ECG examples are shown in Figure 3.18a and b, respectively.

Movement

If a movement sensor (actimeter) is used, move the baby's foot (or limb of attachment) to be sure that motion can be detected. If the signal is unsatisfactory, the sensor must be reapplied or replaced. Different sensors and acquisition systems will produce different looking signals on the recording. The example of movement in Figure 3.19,

ACT, shows a black bar that indicates movement presence and duration on one commercial computerized system.

Position

With the infant supine, verify that a supine reading is recorded. If the reading is not correct, change the sensor orientation until body positions of the baby and the recording signal match. An illustration of one type of position signal is shown in Figure 3.20.

The technician should document these calibration signals and store them during computer data acquisition. A half-hour to an hour should be allotted for adjustments. Rushing at this point is not advised. A shorter recording of high quality is more valuable than a long one with deteriorating signals. All adjustments must be documented on paper tracings, on a checklist (see CHIME checklist in Appendix B), and on the computer screen as appropriate.

PROBLEM WAVEFORM RECOGNITION

During the set-up period and later during the actual recording period, a variety of waveforms will be observed which require documentation or adjustment of filters or electrode derivations, such as changes in the EMG electrode pair, or even require intervention to fix placements.

In some cases, as with motion artifacts, it may be prudent to wait a minute or so to see if the signals improve when the movements or crying have ended. Technician comments should be entered to explain all actions taken during the troubleshooting/signal quality-checking period and during calibrations. Examples of problem waveforms are shown in Figures 3.6, 3.18b and 3.21–3.25. The captions include suggestions for corrective actions.

FROM BEGIN STUDY TO END STUDY

Begin study

When the baby is fed and burped, all sensors are applied and quality signals are being recorded, record 30 s to 1 min of the 50 or 100 µV calibration signals just prior to the epoch that will be designated as 'Begin study' or 'Lights out'. This point should be documented by a comment such as 'Lights out' or

Table 3.5 Collaborative Home Infant Monitoring Evaluation (CHIME) emergency procedure during infant polysomnography

---

Emergency procedure during infant polysomnography

There will be very few instances during the carefully monitored and supervised overnight PSG recordings when clinical interventions will be indicated

If an apnea greater than 20 s in duration occurs, it is advisable to look at the SaO_2 and heart rate. If a downward trend is evident, look at the baby, refraining from stimulating her (him) until:

- Oxygen saturation (SaO_2) is < 85% for > 30 s, or

- Heart rate is < 60 beats/min for at least 10 s

Emergency intervention

- If baby is having a significant clinical event as described above, stimulate the baby by flicking the heels

- If the significant clinical event continues, make sure the airway is patent, reposition and suction if needed, and bag the baby with a few puffs of oxygen (O_2)

- If the perfusion and SaO_2 do not return to previous levels, continue to bag baby and call the appropriate code for physician

- If seizure activity is noted (rather than tremors), verify the electroencephalogram. Check for cyanosis and airway patency. Provide supplemental O_2 to maintain saturation at pre-seizure level. Page the appropriate physician

---

'Begin study'. After this point, there should be explicit procedures for what must be documented and what interventions are permitted.

Documentation

All filter and gain changes, electrode selections and impedances should be documented not only on a technician log or checklist (Appendix B), but also on the actual paper tracing or computer comments screen.

Since time and computer storage may be limited, a system of abbreviations can be most helpful for documentation. The scheme used in the CHIME study is outlined in Appendix D. Elaboration is best made on a checklist or supplemental sheet designed for this purpose. Technician comments entered on the CHIME data acquisition computer appear as text entries in many of the waveform example figures, such as Figure 3.22.

Interventions

All interventions must be documented. In order to preserve the infant's most usual sleep/wake pattern over the course of the recording period, interventions to replace electrodes need to be minimized. Infants can be very sensitive to touching their face/head and checking these electrodes can result in extended crying periods. Unless an essential channel is lost (all EEGs, EOGs or ECG), interventions should wait for a feeding/consoling time. If the infant is fussing, the caregiver should be advised as to consoling procedures. If possible wait a few minutes to see if the infant will return to sleep on his/her own. During feedings, airflow sensors may need to be moved; replacement should not be forgotten.

Emergency interventions

Each laboratory will have its own criteria for what constitutes a medical emergency. Staff must be well trained to recognize the conditions that require observation and documentation only versus immediate intervention or resuscitation. As an example, the emergency procedure used by CHIME is given in Table 3.5.

End study

The criteria for ending a study will vary. For the CHIME study, the basic criterion was a duration of at least 8 h after 'Begin study'. In addition to documenting this point by writing or typing in 'End study' or 'Lights out', one backup technique is to record a 30-s or 1-min period of calibration signals just after 'End study' or 'Lights out'. This calibration, along with the one recorded prior to 'Begin study', serve as 'bookends' around the official recording period. The next step is to test and document the electrode impedances before any electrodes are removed.

At this point, the data acquisition recording can be terminated. If a computerized system is in use and the data backs up automatically it will probably start now. If not, it is important to have a procedure to insure that the data are on a permanent storage medium. Many options are available for computer-assisted systems; for example, ZIP disks, CDs and optical disks.

Once the recording has ended, the staff can enter the sleep room and begin to remove the sensors. The baby can be washed gently to remove excess gel and dressed to return to the nursery or home. Any exit paperwork can be completed. Finally, all sensors must be cleaned in preparation for the next IPSG. Some laboratories may want to consider implementing a quality review of the recording to give feedback to the staff that did the recording. A sample of the procedure CHIME developed is in Appendix E. It may be prudent to review the recording and technician remarks the morning the IPSG ends. Any suspicious or clearly significant activity or events can be flagged for immediate review and follow-up even if the actual scoring has not been started.

REFERENCES

1. American Medical Association. *Current Procedural Terminology CPT 2002*, 4th edn. Chicago: AMA Press, 2001

2. American Thoracic Society. Standards and indications for cardiopulmonary sleep studies in children. *Am J Res Crit Care Med* 1996;53:866–78

3. American Academy of Pediatrics. Clinical practice guidelines: diagnosis and management of childhood obstructive sleep apnea syndrome. *Pediatrics* 2002;109:704–12

4. American Academy of Pediatrics. Technical Report: diagnosis and management of childhood obstructive sleep apnea syndrome. *Pediatrics* 2002;109:1–20

5. Jasper HH. The ten twenty electrode system of the International Federation. *Electroencephalogr Clin Neurophysiol* 1985;10:371–5

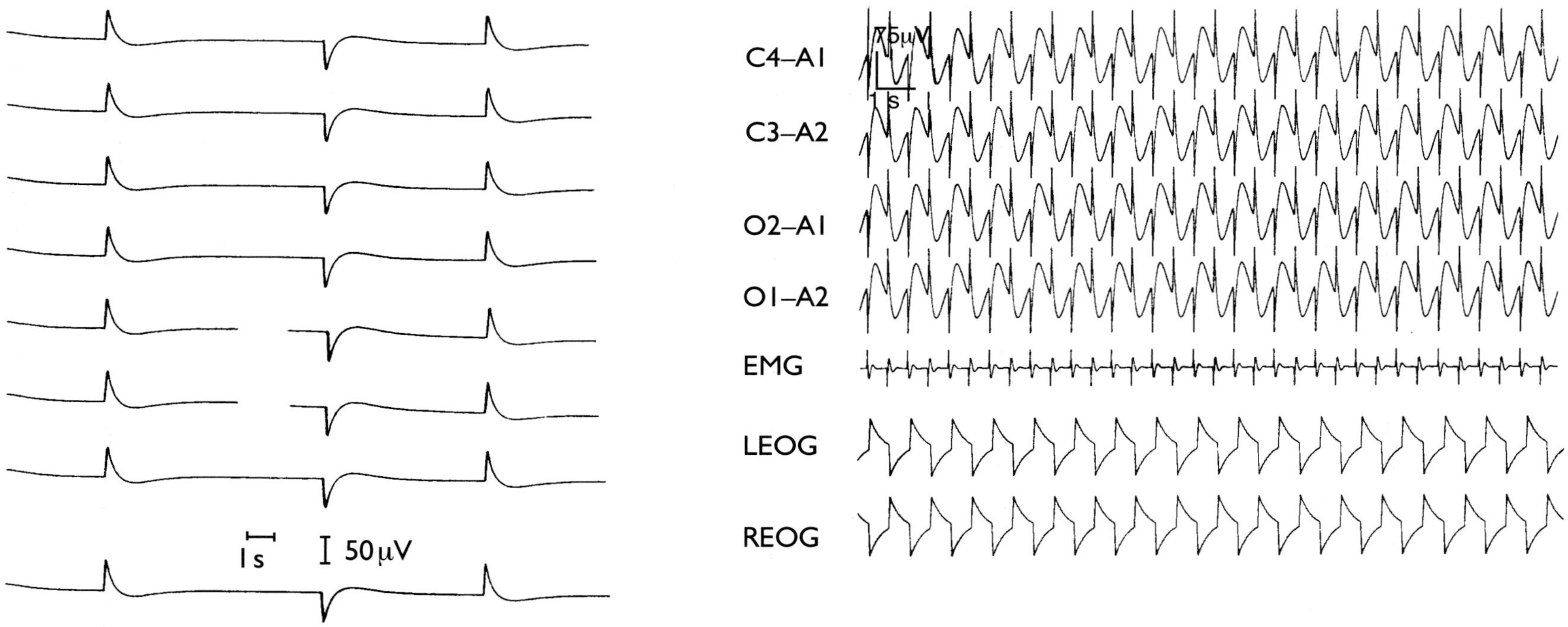

Figure 3.1 Pre-polysomnogram calibration of AC channel amplifiers. a, 50 μV calibration signal on all channels at the same filter settings; b, variations in 100 μV calibration signals due to different filter settings for electroencephalogram (EEG; C4–A1 to O1–A2), electromyogram (EMG) and electrooculogram (EOG)

a

Low-frequency filter	0.3 Hz	
High-frequency filter	20 Hz	
Sensitivity	50 μV/cm	
60 Hz off		

b

EEG	Low-frequency filter	1.0 Hz
	High-frequency filter	40 Hz
EMG	Low-frequency filter	5.0 Hz
	High-frequency filter	45 Hz
EOG	Low-frequency filter	0.3 Hz
	High-frequency filter	40 Hz
Sensitivity		100 μV/cm
60 Hz notch filter on		

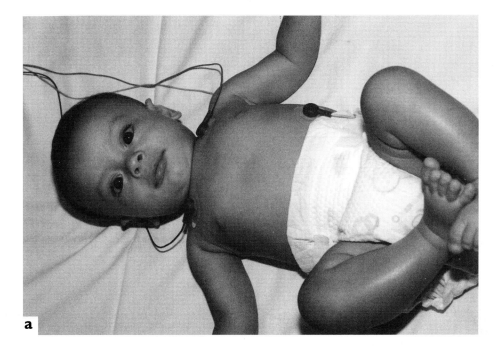

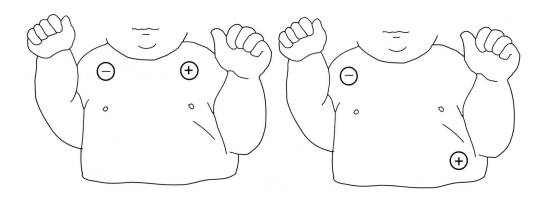

Lead 1   Lead 2

b

Figure 3.2 a, Electrocardiogram sensor placement and b, schematic of placements for modified Lead 1 and 2. The (-) and (+) electrodes reflect the polarity of the electrical output of the heartbeat. Typically, the polarity is established so that the R-wave deflection is upwards

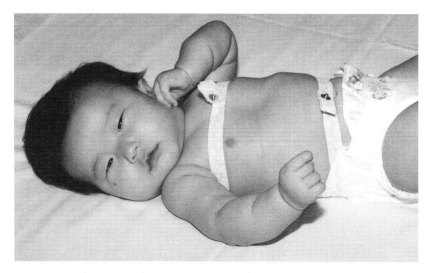

Figure 3.3 Placement of respiratory motion bands around the rib cage above the nipple line and the abdomen near the umbilicus

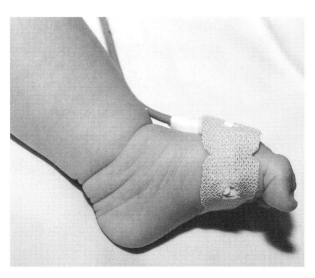

Figure 3.4 Placement of the oximeter sensor on the foot

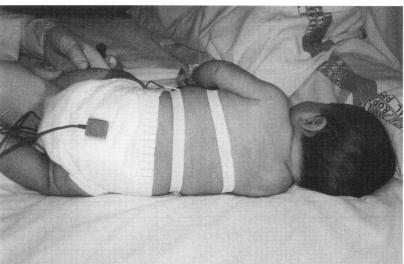

Figure 3.5 Position sensor placement on the back of the diaper taped in the direction that produces a supine deflection when the infant is supine. Photograph courtesy of Straub Clinic & Hospital

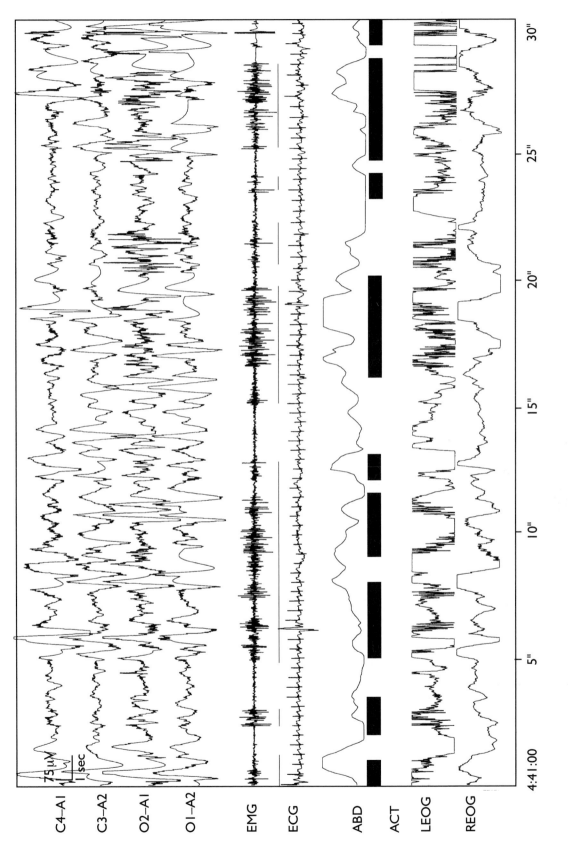

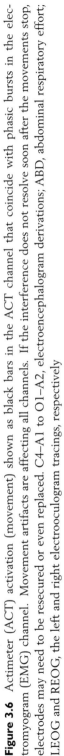

Figure 3.6 Actimeter (ACT) activation (movement) shown as black bars in the ACT channel that coincide with phasic bursts in the electromyogram (EMG) channel. Movement artifacts are affecting all channels. If the interference does not resolve soon after the movements stop, electrodes may need to be rescued or even replaced. C4–A1 to O1–A2, electroencephalogram derivations; ABD, abdominal respiratory effort; LEOG and REOG, the left and right electrooculogram tracings, respectively

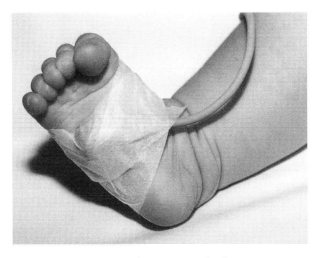

Figure 3.7 Actimeter placement on the foot

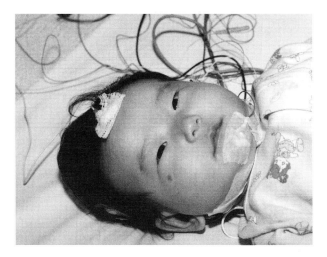

Figure 3.8 Digastric (submental) electromyogram electrode placement sites: one electrode on the point of the chin and two on the submental area under the chin. Electrodes under the chin should be placed as far back as possible

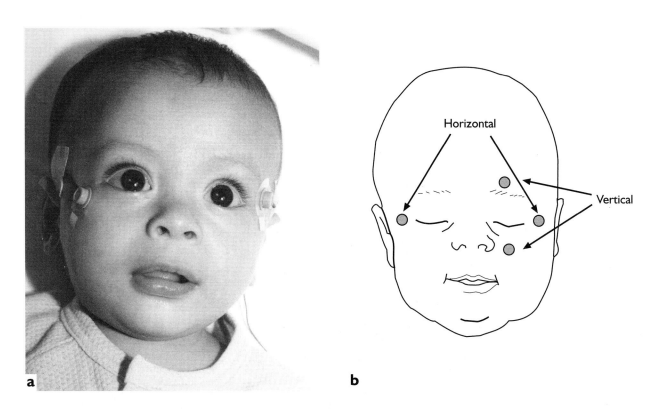

Figure 3.9 a, Electrooculogram (EOG) electrode placements with the left EOG out from and above the outer canthus of the left eye and the right EOG out from and below the outer canthus of the right eye. For a two-channel recording, each eye lead is referred to the same reference site, e.g. the left mastoid (M1). b, Schematic of the vertical and horizontal electrode placement sites for two-channel EOG recordings. The horizontal leads can also be referred to each other to produce a single-channel left and right outer canthus (LOC to ROC) recording

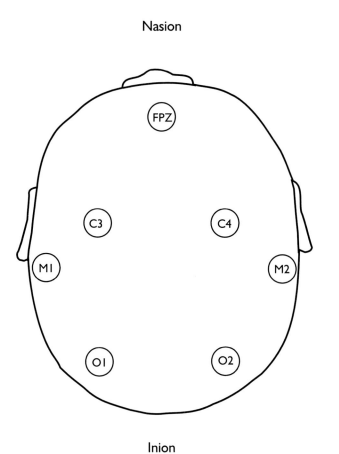

Nasion

Inion

Figure 3.10 Infant electroencephalogram electrode placement sites: left and right central (C3 and C4), left and right occipital (O1 and O2), inactive reference sites on the left and right bony mastoid processes (M1 and M2), also referred to as A1 and A2, and the patient ground electrode on the mid-forehead (FPZ)

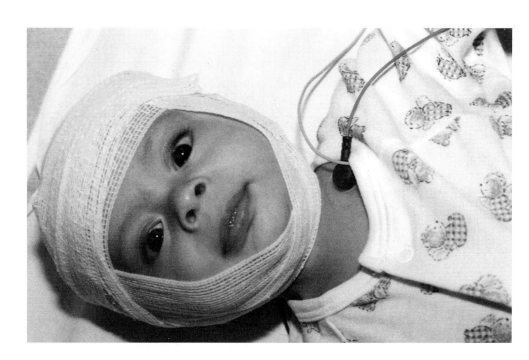

Figure 3.11 Head wrap used to secure electrodes during infant polysomnography

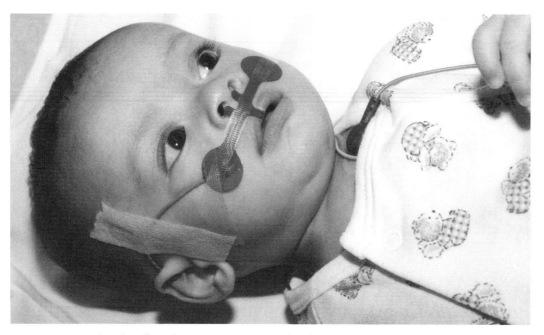

Figure 3.12 Nasal/oral airflow thermistor/thermocouple placement in front of, but not touching the nares, mouth or face

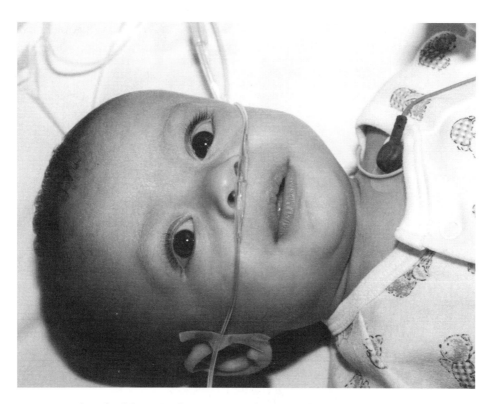

Figure 3.13 Expired, end-tidal CO_2 tubing or, as in this example, nasal cannula, placement into the nares

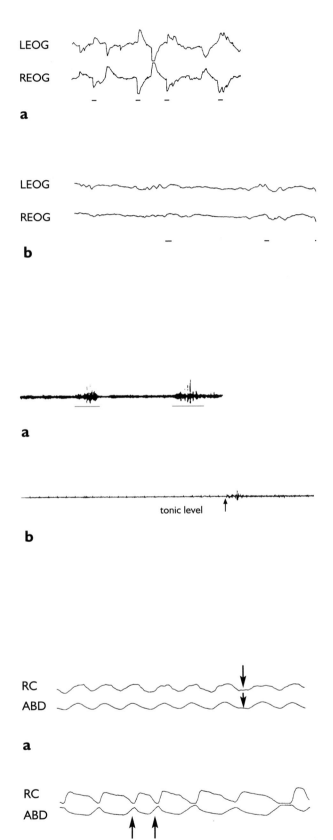

a

b

Figure 3.14 a, Opposite polarity awake rapid eye movements. Left electrooculogram (LEOG) deflections are 'up' and right EOG (REOG) deflections are 'down' (see underlines). b, Same polarity eye movements are indicated by the underlines

a

b

Figure 3.15 a, Submental electromyogram (EMG) with sucking bursts (underlined); b, minimal tonic level during active sleep is followed by a phasic burst (starting at the arrow) and then a sustained increase in the tonic level

a

b

Figure 3.16 a, Synchronous respiratory effort in rib cage (RC) and abdomen (ABD) where inspiration produces upward deflections in both channels (see arrows). b, Out-of-phase or paradoxical effort in RC and ABD, where inspiration is an upward deflection in RC and a downward deflection in ABD (see arrows)

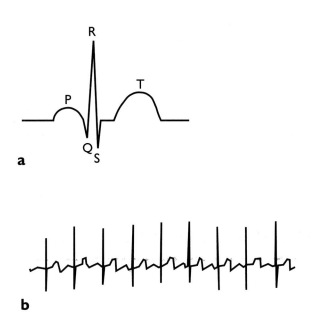

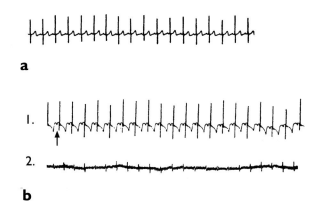

a

1.

2.

b

Figure 3.18 a, Optimal electrocardiogram (ECG) signals. b, Poor ECG complex recordings: reversed polarity as indicated by the downward deflection of the P-wave (1; see arrow); 60-Hz noise (wide dark band) that obscures the low-amplitude ECG complex (2)

Figure 3.17 a, Stylized illustration of the normal electrocardiogram (ECG) PQRST waves. b, A sample of an ECG tracing from an infant polysomnogram

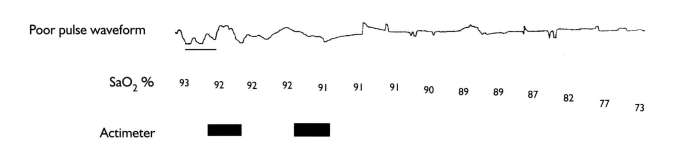

Poor pulse waveform

SaO$_2$ % 93 92 92 92 91 91 91 90 89 89 87 82 77 73

Actimeter

Figure 3.19 Actimeter movement sensor indicator where movement presence and duration are shown as a black bar. Movement is confirmed by the loss of the pulse (two pulses are underlined) in the pulse waveform signal. After the loss of pulse signals, oxygen saturation (SaO$_2$) percent values are not reliable

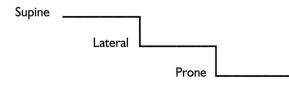

Figure 3.20 Illustration of a position sensor recording output where changes in signal level denote the position detected by the sensor

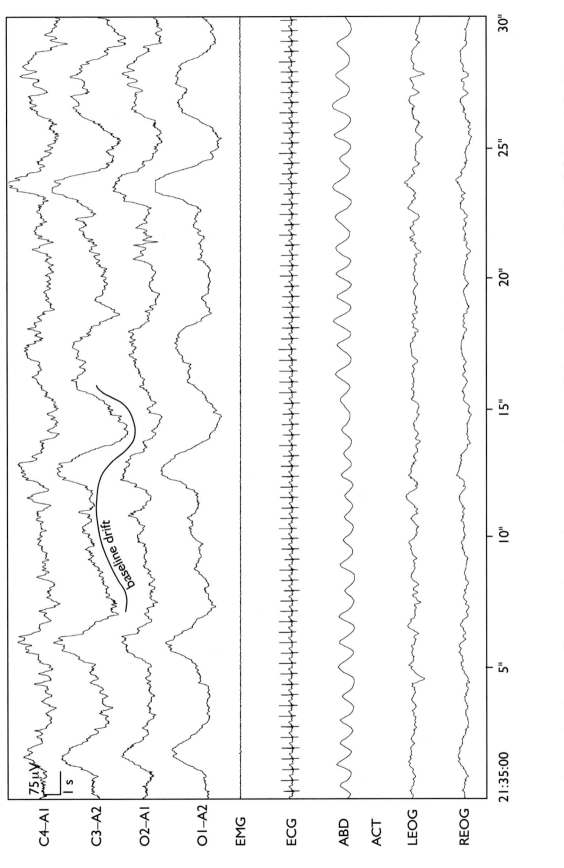

Figure 3.21 A low-frequency filter setting that is too low, creating an electroencephalogram (C4–A1 to O1–A2) baseline drift (see underline). To stabilize the baseline, the filter setting should be increased. EMG, submental electromyogram; ECG, electrocardiogram; ABD, abdominal respiration; ACT, actimeter; LEOG and REOG, left and right electrooculogram, respectively

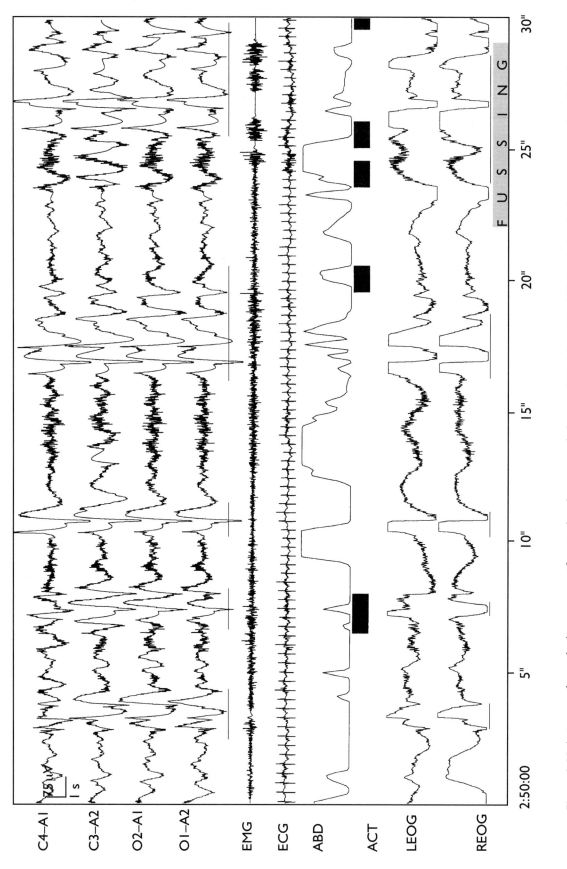

Figure 3.22 Active awake with slow-wave artifact in the electroencephalogram (C4–A1 to O1–A2) (underlined) that is associated with high-voltage eye movements (left and right electrooculogram (LEOG and REOG; underlined) and body movements shown by the black actimeter (ACT) bars. Wait for the infant to quiet or fall asleep. The movement-related artifacts should resolve spontaneously. EMG, submental electromyogram; ECG, electrocardiogram; ABD, abdominal respiration

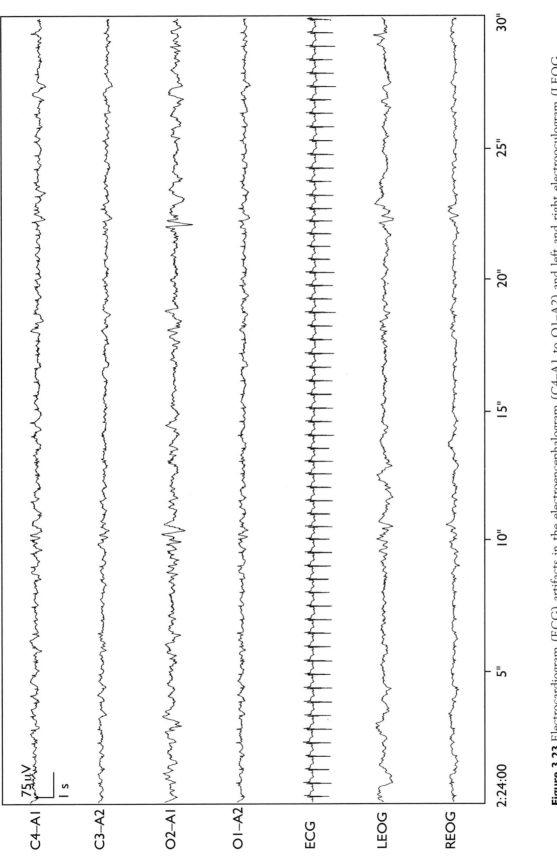

Figure 3.23 Electrocardiogram (ECG) artifacts in the electroencephalogram (C4–A1 to O1–A2) and left and right electrooculogram (LEOG, REOG, respectively) appearing as sharp spikes congruent with the ECG R-waves. Re-referencing A1 and A2 to A1 + A2 should reduce or eliminate these ECG spikes. If the EOGs are not referenced to the mastoids, you may decide to tolerate these artifacts or attempt to eliminate them by moving the electrode sites slightly

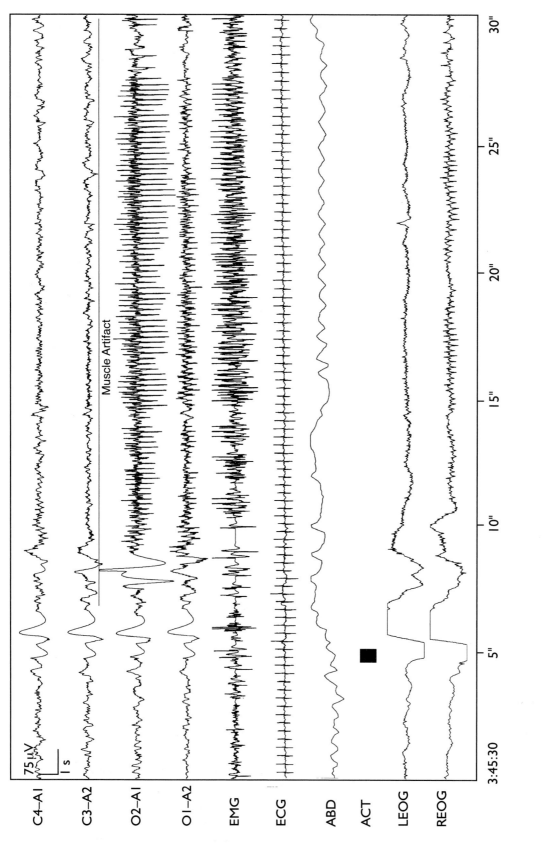

Figure 3.24 Muscle artifact in the electromyogram (EMG) that appears in varying amplitudes in the electroencephalogram (C4–A1 to O1–A2) and left and right electrooculogram (LEOG, REOG, respectively). If this artifact does not clear spontaneously after the baby is quiet, another EMG electrode combination should be tried. If this does not resolve the problem, impedance on electrodes must be obtained, and at the earliest opportunity, high-impedance leads must be checked and resecured, or replaced if necessary. ABD, abdominal respiration; ACT, actimeter

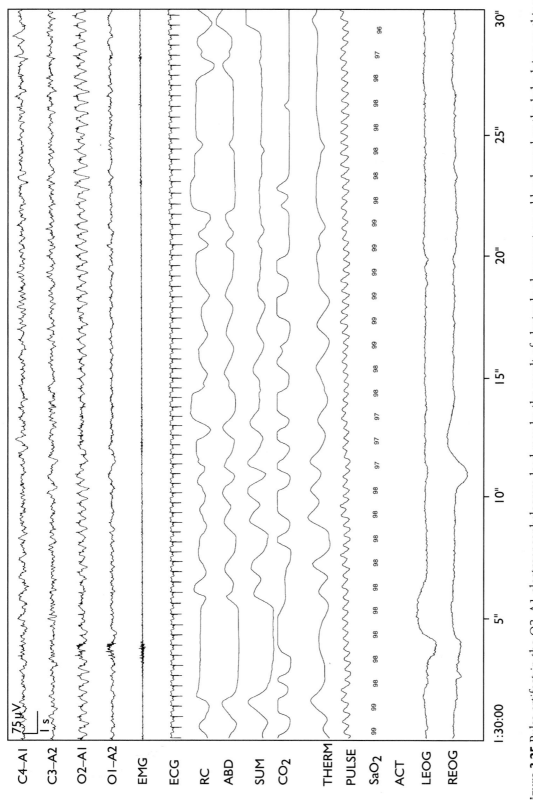

Figure 3.25 Pulse artifact in the O2–A1 electroencephalogram lead may be the result of electrode placement on a blood vessel or the baby lying on this electrode. If scoring cannot be completed from the other electroencephalogram (C4–A1; C3–A2; O1–A2) channels, at the earliest feeding or awake period remove the electrode and reposition it in the right occipital area where it does not pick up a pulse. To eliminate electrocardiogram (ECG) artifacts present in all EEG channels, join the A1 and A2 reference electrodes instead of using A1 or A2 alone. EMG, electromyogram; RC, rib cage; ABD, abdominal respiration; SUM, weighted sum of RC and ABD; CO$_2$, end-tidal CO$_2$; THERM, nasal/oral thermistor; PULSE, the oximeter pulse waveform; SaO$_2$, oxygen saturation percent values; ACT, actimeter; LEOG and REOG, left and right electrooculogram, respectively

4

Infant polysomnography scoring procedures

This Chapter covers the identification and scoring of awake and sleep states for infants < 3 months of age post-term, sleep stages for infants ≥ 3 months of age post-term, transient arousal, cardiorespiratory events and final summary reports.

WAKE STATE RECOGNITION

One of the major differences between scoring PSGs in older children and adults and IPSGs is the inability to discern infant awake periods based on EEG, EMG and eye movement patterns. Although there may be EEG waveforms in the alpha range (8–13 Hz), the adult-type alpha that is present in the awake-eyes closed state and disappears with eye opening is not regularly observed in infants[1-5]. Therefore, most infant scoring guidelines[6-10] rely on direct observation of the infant to determine the awake state. The CHIME protocol defined awake periods as those marked by eyes open, crying periods, feeding and diapering intervention. Technician documentation of the beginning and end of periods designated as 'awake' is critical to the correct interpretation of the IPSG because scoring of sleep state or stage applies only to sleep epochs. A clear definition of awake periods is also important for the identification of arousals and sleep-related cardiorespiratory events. To illustrate awake tracings, that is, those documented by observations according to the above criteria, examples of quiet awake and active awake periods are shown in Figures 4.1–4.3. Transition from wake to sleep with documentation about wake start and stop times is shown in Figure 4.4. The technician should document what he/she observes, e.g. 'eyes open' rather than simply 'awake'.

All the examples of awake, sleep state and sleep stage display only the primary sleep scoring channels. Display of only these channels on computer monitors enhances the definition of each parameter. CHIME used the following alternate montage display for sleep state and stage scoring: EEG (C4–A1, C3–A2, O2–A1, O1–A2), submental EMG, ECG, abdominal respiratory effort (ABD), the movement sensor (actimeter, ACT), eye movement (LEOG and REOG) and technician comments.

SLEEP STATE IDENTIFICATION

Although several approaches have been espoused for sleep state recognition in pre-term[11], term[6] and infants up to 6 months post-term[8,12], this Atlas was derived from CHIME study procedures that applied the standards developed by Anders and colleagues[6] for full-term newborns to this entire age range[12]. Modifications to the system of Anders and colleagues[6] may be necessary to extend the procedures from the preterm period to the post-term period through 6 months post term. It has been recognized that by 6 weeks to 3 months post-term[8,12], the adult sleep stage scoring system of Rechtschaffen and Kales[13] begins to be more consistent with the EEG at this age and is described in the sleep stage determination section that follows sleep state. Sleep state identification was based on the individual assessment of the following physiological parameters: EEG, EOG, EMG, respiration, that is abdominal effort (ABD), the direct (ACT) and indirect indications of body movements and comments or vocalizations (VOC).

Directions for scoring each of these parameters follows the identification section.

EEG

Infant EEG is distinctive with patterns changing as the infant matures. The importance of these changes warrants a detailed discussion of the EEG itself in terms of frequency components or bands along with patterns and features that define maturational changes. Then, the particular EEG patterns associated with sleep state recognition are defined in the 'EEG as a scoring parameter' section and examples presented in the section on sleep state scoring. Examples of the EEG frequencies typically found in the IPSG are depicted in Figure 4.5. The alpha-frequency band (8–13 Hz) is included because frequencies in this range can be observed[4] although they do not necessarily correspond to the awake state. Other EEG features present in this age group include spindles that develop around 6 weeks post-term[14] (Figure 4.6). Detailed descriptions of EEG in normal and abnormal infants can be found in the atlases of Sheldon and associates[15], Stockard-Pope and colleagues[16] and in Niedermeyer[5].

Spindle development

Sleep spindle frequencies are in the range of 12–14 Hz in adults but in infants may be in the 9–11 Hz range. Faster frequencies (13–15 Hz) can appear as rudimentary or pre-spindles at approximately term conceptional age[17] (Figure 4.6a). Spindle activity becomes more prominent around 6 weeks post-term and may be asynchronous between the right and left hemispheres[14] (Figure 4.6b). After 52 weeks' conceptional age, spindles are expected to be present and become part of more adult-appearing sleep patterns that can begin to define Stage 2 or NREM sleep (see section on sleep stages; Figure 4.6c). Other EEG features in infants <6 months adjusted age include: sharp transients[5] (Figure 4.7a), sharp components in slow wave bursts[5] (Figure 4.7b), delta-brush[16] (Figure 4.7c) and spontaneous K-complexes[18] (Figure 4.7d). The maturational course of the EEG during awake periods and sleep in infants through 6 months' adjusted age is summarized in Figure 4.8[19]. A more extensive table of maturational features from prematurity through adolescence can be found in Niedermeyer[5].

EEG as a state scoring parameter

Using the EEG frequency bands and patterns presented previously, along with certain age-specific patterns, Anders and colleagues[6] incorporated the EEG into their sleep state scoring procedures. When scoring sleep state, however, EEG is only one of several parameters that together comprise the final state determination; these include EEG, EOG, submental EMG, respiratory rate regularity and movements. The following section describes the characteristics of each parameter evaluated for non-wake, that is, sleep epochs, from 'Begin study' to 'End study'. The first parameter presented here is the EEG.

The four primary EEG state-related patterns as described by Anders and colleagues[6] are described in Figure 4.9 and paired with waveform examples of each pattern. As noted earlier, in the CHIME study, these definitions were applied to infants across the sampled age groups[20]. This procedure was established to provide for standardization across the research study clinical sites and also to facilitate comparisons between the age groups. This approach may not be desirable in every case. For scoring purposes the EEG pattern that occupies > 50% of an epoch can be assigned a code for that epoch. This code will then become a part of the state scoring process described in the section on sleep state determination. Because shifts in the EEG may occur between or across epochs, it may be prudent to consider the EEG patterns prior to and after a particular epoch when assigning the epoch code.

EOG

Eye movements are an important variable in state determination as rapid eye movements (REMs) are associated with the active sleep (AS) state[6,21–23]. The presence or absence of one or more REMs determines eye movement coding in an epoch. This decision requires two EOG channels that produce synchronized oppositional deflections (Figure 4.10). In very young infants, REMs may not exceed background variations with sufficient amplitude to make identification easy. REMs that occur during movement periods, crying or artifacts are not counted.

EMG

The submental EMG is another indicator that is a very useful parameter for discriminating sleep stages in older children and adults but has had variable success in differentiating sleep states in infants[24-26]. The younger the infant the more difficult it is to see differences in the tonic or baseline EMG. Phasic EMG bursts are not considered in this phase of parameter coding. If variation in the submental tonic level cannot be discerned throughout the IPSG, then this variable should be deleted from the parameters used in sleep state coding. An epoch is classified as high (elevated) or low EMG based on whichever level occupies at least 50% of an epoch (Figure 4.11a and b).

Respiration

Regularity of respiratory effort is the determining factor for coding respiration as it relates to sleep state[6]. Most commonly, this measurement is based on the waveform pattern of respiratory effort as it can be measured most consistently in young infants. CHIME used the abdominal effort tracing as the primary respiratory sleep state scoring channel. The determination of regularity is somewhat controversial as frequency characteristics can vary with age[27], particularly in the very young, premature infant. One method suggested by Anders and colleagues[6] was to consider the difference in rate between the shortest and longest rate. This is not always easy to determine but peak-to-peak distances can be calculated and converted to breaths per minute (Figure 4.12). If the difference between the shortest and longest values is greater than 20, then the epoch would be considered to have irregular respiration. If the difference is less than 20, the epoch would be considered to be regular. When identifying the shortest and longest peak-to-peak breath intervals, periods of movement artifacts and pauses of more than 3-s duration should be excluded. Computer-assisted scoring system measurement tools are very useful in making these calculations.

Movements

Movements are an important component in defining infant sleep state[6,28,29]. Presence or absence of movements should be documented by direct observation but can also be supplemented by sensors such as actimeters that mark the recording when movements occur (Figure 4.13). Indirect measures of movement can be observed in movement-related artifacts such as those seen in a pulse oximeter waveform, the ECG, phasic bursts in the submental EMG or blocking of the EEG. Examples of these indirect measures are shown in Figure 4.14. Phasic activity such as mouthing, startles and sucking that can occur in quiet sleep (QS) should not be considered as movement *per se*. An epoch is considered to have movement if any movement at all (except as noted) is recorded. On occasion, epochs that are considered part of the sleep time may be obscured by body movements making it impossible to determine parameter codes. In these cases, the epoch should not be scored for sleep state, but it could be designated by a special code such as movement time. Other techniques for handling these unscorable epochs are in the sleep state determination section.

The final process in determining a sleep state for each epoch is to form combinations of the individual parameter codes for that epoch. This process is described in the following section.

SLEEP STATE DETERMINATION

Once the individual parameter attributes are determined, those characteristics identified with QS and AS are counted[6] (Table 4.1). The final state assigned is based on whether the majority of attributes or patterns are QS, AS or neither. If neither QS nor AS can be assigned, then indeterminate sleep (IS) is assigned to this epoch. Awake is scored regardless of the individual parameters as it is based on observer comments (eyes open, crying, feeding, etc.). Awake examples are presented in Figures 4.1–4.3. One method of determining whether an epoch will be considered QS or AS[6,30] is to observe if 5/5 of the parameters are associated with QS. If so, the epoch will be coded as QS. Some variation is possible at this point. For example, requiring 5/5 may be considered too stringent and only 4/5 QS parameters are required to code the epoch as QS. If the EMG is rejected from the evaluation due to lack of variation in the tonic level then the state decision would have a denominator of 4 and a requirement of 4/4 or 3/4. The same process applies to AS; if 5/5 or 4/5 codes are AS codes, then the epoch is considered

Table 4.1 Parameter codes associated with quiet sleep (QS) and active sleep (AS). Adapted from reference 6

State	Individual parameters	
QS	EEG	high voltage slow, tracé alternant or mixed
	EOG	no REMs
	EMG	high
	RESP	regular
	BM	absent (except mouthing, sucking)
AS	EEG	low voltage irregular, mixed
	EOG	one or more REMs
	EMG	low
	RESP	irregular
	BM	present

EEG, electroencephalogram; EOG, electrooculogram; EMG, submental electromyogram; RESP, abdominal respiratory motion; BM, body movements; REM, rapid eye movement

as AS. Some epochs will yield codes that do not meet QS or AS criteria. For example, there may be three QS and two AS codes or vice versa. In these cases, the epoch will be considered to reflect IS. Figures 4.15–4.24 show IPSG 30-s epochs that illustrate the individual parameter characteristics given in Table 4.1 and the final sleep state determined by the combination of these characteristics.

Each laboratory should determine if they will assign a state to each individual epoch or if they want to employ some form of smoothing procedure. For example, if one epoch of another state (often IS or possibly movement time) interrupts an ongoing period of another sleep state, this discrepant epoch may be scored the same as the surrounding states. Another possibility is to consider longer time periods, such as 1-min periods, as an epoch[31].

RELIABILITY OF SLEEP STATE CODING

Before any scoring system is accepted by a sleep laboratory the staff who score the tracings should be well-educated in the rules and methods selected. As a part of the training and competency procedures, reliability between all potential scorers should be tested and retraining implemented until sufficient reliability has been achieved[20]. Periodic reliability testing should be implemented and new scorers must

establish reliability. The IPSG reliability study conducted for the CHIME IPSG dataset demonstrated that substantial levels of agreement can be obtained for sleep parameters and states in the CHIME study age range[20].

The CHIME study elected to use the same sleep state scoring method[20] across all conceptional ages that were included in their research design in order to have comparative data for all study infants. Other investigators and clinicians, however, have applied alternative scoring methods for infants beyond approximately 52 weeks' conceptional age. These methods typically reflect some modification of adult scoring methods such as those of Rechtschaffen and Kales[13]. In fact, the term sleep stage is frequently used from this early age on and this method of scoring of stages is described in the following section.

SLEEP STAGE DETERMINATION

It has been shown that at approximately 52 weeks' conceptional age, the EEG begins to take on a more 'adult' look in QS[12,32–35]. For this reason, it becomes increasingly possible to apply adult scoring methods such as Rechtschaffen and Kales[13] and Anders and colleagues[36] or modifications of adult criteria[8,32] as the conceptional age increases. Other investigators have designated 6 months post-term as the point where adult scoring methods are appropriate[37].

The period between 43 and 52 weeks' conceptional age reflects the transition from newborn full-term sleep patterns toward adult patterns. As noted earlier, some of the hallmarks of adult sleep, such as K-complexes, do not appear until 5–7 months post-term. Waking alpha does not begin to appear until 1–3 years of age and the alpha-frequency band may be slower than in adults, between 6–7 Hz rather than 8–13 Hz. Since the awake state still cannot be defined by alpha EEG frequencies in the eyes-closed condition, the infant state reliance on behavioral criteria must continue to be applied. If an infant around 1 year or more demonstrates sufficient alpha then it can be incorporated into the wake stage identification for that infant.

At the early ages where the transition from state to stage occurs, modifications such as the scheme of Guilleminault and Souquet[32] provide a means to use stage characteristics even when all the components such as spindles may not be present. In contrast to the individual parameter method for state identification, stages are based primarily on the EEG, EOG and submental EMG[13]. One scheme for sleep stage determination in this age group[13] is given in Table 4.2. Figures 4.25–4.32 show epochs of stages based on the definitions in Table 4.2.

Guilleminault and Souquet[8,32] were of the opinion that the method of Anders and colleagues[6] did not take advantage of all the information available in the EEG of older infants and proposed a two-phase system that applies one set of criteria from 3 to 6 months and another from 6 months on. Their system is outlined in Table 4.3.

Table 4.2 Adult sleep stage scoring criteria applied to CHIME infant polysomnograms after 46 weeks' conceptional age. Modified from reference 13

Stage	Criteria
Wake	infant criteria for awake were applied and include eyes open, crying, caregiver intervention or movement artifacts occupying more than 50% of an epoch and lasting longer than two consecutive epochs. For example, from eyes open (EO) to eyes closed (EC) annotation
Stage 1	relatively low-voltage, mixed-frequency EEG, predominantly 2–7 Hz, of up to 75 μV, occurring in irregularly spaced bursts during the latter portions of the stage. Vertex sharp waves up to 200 μV may be present. Absolute absence of K-complexes and sleep spindles. Spindles of 12–14 Hz of less than 0.5-s duration may be present. Eye movements are slow and of several seconds duration; rapid eye movements (REMs) are absent
Stage 2	sleep spindles and/or K-complexes are present. Sleep spindles must be at least 0.5-s duration with six to seven distinct waves in the 0.5-s period. High-voltage, slow EEG pattern does not occupy more than 20% of the epoch. If < 3 min of the record that could ordinarily meet the criteria for Stage 1 intervene between sleep spindles or K-complexes, these epochs are scored as Stage 2 if there is no movement arousal or EMG increase during the interval. If the interval is ≥ 3 min, score as Stage 1. If movement arousals or EMG increases occur, the portion prior is Stage 2 and that after is Stage 1 until Stage 2 spindle or K-complex criteria are met
Stage 3	epoch in which at least 20% but not more than 50% of the EEG consists of ≤ 2 Hz waves with peak-to-peak amplitudes of > 75 μV. Sleep spindles may or may not be present
Stage 4	epoch in which > 50% of the EEG is 2 Hz or slower with peak-to-peak amplitudes > 75 μV. Sleep spindles may or may not be present
Stage REM	defined by the concomitant appearance of relatively low-voltage, mixed-frequency EEG and episodic REMs. EEG resembles Stage 1. Distinctive 'saw-tooth' waves frequently, but not always, appear with REM bursts. There is an absolute absence of sleep spindles and K-complexes. Stage REM should not be scored in the presence of *relatively* elevated tonic submental EMG

EEG, electroencephalogram; EMG, submental electromyogram

Table 4.3   Sleep stage scoring methods of Guilleminault and Souquet[31] for infants 3–6 months post-term. Adapted from reference 31 with permission

3 months	6 months (4.5 weeks – 1 year of age)
Wakefulness	*Wakefulness*
EEG mixed frequency, no delta (< 75 µV) EOG eye movements EMG high amplitude	same as at 3 months
	Stage 1

Stage 1–2 (combined)	EEG predominance of theta
	               absence of spindles
	               absence of delta (> 150 µV)

EEG   predominance of theta
         presence or absence of spindles
         less than 20% delta (> 150 µV)/epoch
EOG   possible rolling eye movements
EMG   variable
	EOG possible rolling eye movements
	EMG variable

	Stage 2
Stage 3–4 (combined)	EEG predominance of theta presence of spindles < 20% delta (> 150 µV)/epoch
EEG at least 20% delta (> 150 µV)/epoch EOG no eye movements EMG variable	EOG no eye movement EMG variable
	Stage 3–4
Stage REM EEG predominance of theta EOG rapid eye movements EMG variable	same as for 3 months
	Stage REM
	same as for 3 months except the infant is quieter at this age

EEG, electroencephalogram; EOG, electrooculogram; EMG, submental electromyogram; REM, rapid eye movement

SMOOTHING OF SLEEP STATE/STAGE SCORING RESULTS

Sleep architecture is a term applied to the graphic representation of changes in sleep and wake states over the course of a recording period. Wide variability in state can be noted from one epoch to another, and there is some controversy whether this is a result of scoring artifacts or infant physiological lability. One technique that can be applied to the discrete epoch data that reduces, or smoothes over, some of the transient variations, is referred to as smoothing. Smoothing itself can be affected by a number of variables such as epoch length and the smoothing window (number of epochs smoothed). An example of how smoothing changes the sleep architecture representation is shown in Figure 4.33. Figure 4.33 illustrates the progression from states assigned to each 30-s epoch and no smoothing to a 1-min epoch length and a five-epoch smoothing window.

AROUSALS DURING SLEEP

In the analysis of sleep, the term arousal is applied to changes from sleep states or stages to wakefulness or EEG activity similar to the awake state[13,38,39]. The recognition of arousals and the circumstances of their occurrence are considered to have fundamental biological/physiological significance[40,41] and clinical significance[42–49]. Long recordings such as all-night IPSG will include numerous state changes or transitions with long periods of waking for feeding and diaper changes. In addition to these awakenings, state transitions occur frequently as sleep cycles are shorter than in adults, that is, one AS/QS cycle occurs every 50–60 min through 3 months of age with about 50% of the night in AS and 50% in QS[50]. These state changes and transitional periods often begin with 'transient' arousals.

There is a dearth of systematic data on infant arousals. A representative summary of published articles[51] suggests that this situation may be due, in part, to the existing diversity in the definition and the measurement of arousals. Most of these studies, nonetheless, assume the same contextual background implied in the definition of arousal which, in its most generic sense as a transitive verb, is 'to awake from or as if from asleep'[52]. The operational definitions and assessments of arousal in these studies show several 'gold standards' generally based on electrophysiological and/or behavioral criteria to describe functional status along the sleep–wake continuum.

The approach described here defines transient arousals primarily in terms of EEG changes, that is, as electrocortical arousals, following the guidelines proposed in 1992 by the American Sleep Disorders Association (ASDA) Atlas Task Force[53]. Although developed for use with adult sleep studies, the Atlas Task Force criteria for arousals[53] have been modified for IPSGs[51]. Intensive training of IPSG scorers has demonstrated that reliable identification of arousals based on application of these rules is feasible. The Atlas Task Force[53] defined arousal in terms of EEG changes, that is, 'An EEG arousal is an abrupt shift in EEG frequency, which may include theta, alpha and/or other frequencies greater than 16 Hz but not spindles' (p.174). To be included in this definition, the EEG changes should be readily identified as periodic phenomena that disrupt sleep.

Arousals can also be classified in terms of their association with external events or internal stimuli. Arousals that occur in the absence of any discernible stimulus can be classified as 'spontaneous'. The decision of what constitutes a 'discernible' stimulus will depend on the variables monitored and decisions of each laboratory as to definitions of the stimuli. For example, respiratory events that are typically scored for PSGs may be easier to measure with well-understood guidelines but the same may not be true for heart rate or other alterations in the recorded variables. In addition, there must be a critical evaluation of the relationship of proposed stimuli to the arousal. This process differs from the typical PSG task of measuring or tabulating arousals that occur after respiratory events. Although transient EEG arousals can be identified from EEG channels alone, other channels may be added to the scoring montage to allow detection of arousal-associated movements, for example, apneas and sighs. Each laboratory must determine its own specific scoring procedures.

In the CHIME study, sleep states were scored prior to identifying arousals[51]. An alternate montage was selected to evaluate arousals and included the following parameters: EEG (C4–A1; C3–A2; O2–A1; O1–A2), EMG, ECG, SUM, CO_2, thermistor (THERM), pulse waveform (PULSE), SaO_2, actimeter (ACT), LEOG, REOG and comments. SUM is the weighted sum of the rib cage and abdomen signals and is proportional to tidal volume. The CHIME-modified Atlas Task Force EEG arousal definition and scoring rules with italicized modifications[51] are listed below:

Definitions and scoring rules

- Subjects must be asleep, defined as 10 or more continuous seconds of any sleep *state*, before an EEG arousal can be scored (Figure 4.34)

- *Wake periods are defined by technician annotation of eyes open, crying, caregiving intervention, or movement artifact occupying more than 50% of an epoch and lasting greater than two consecutive epochs* (Figure 4.35). *If the arousal proceeds to wake, then the wake epochs that include at least 10 s of sleep may be included in arousal scoring; otherwise, wake epochs would be excluded*

- A minimum of 10 s of continuous intervening sleep is necessary to score a second arousal. When the duration between two arousals is < 10 s then the arousals and the duration between are considered as one arousal (Figure 4.36)

- The EEG frequency shift must be 3 s or greater in duration to be scored as an arousal. *Shifts of > 2.5 s were rounded up to 3 s.* An example of an arousal that does not meet the scoring criteria is shown in Figure 4.37

- Arousals in *quiet sleep and indeterminate sleep* may occur without concurrent increases in submental EMG amplitude

- Arousals are scored in *active sleep* only when accompanied by concurrent increases in submental EMG amplitude (Figure 4.38). Therefore, the EEG arousal (starting at the arrow) in Figure 4.38 could not be scored

- Arousals cannot be scored based on changes in submental EMG amplitude alone (Figure 4.39)

- Artifacts, K-complexes and delta waves are not scored as arousals unless accompanied by an EEG frequency shift (as previously defined) in at least one derivation. If such activity precedes an EEG frequency shift, it is not included in reaching the 3-s duration criterion. When occurring within the EEG frequency shift, artifacts or delta-wave activity can be included in meeting the duration criterion (Figure 4.40)

- The occurrence of pen blocking artifacts should be included in an arousal only if an EEG arousal pattern is contiguous. The pen blocking event can be included in reaching the duration criterion (Figure 4.41)

- Non-concurrent, but contiguous EEG and EMG changes, which are individually less than 3 s but together greater than 3 s in duration are not scored as arousals

- Intrusion of alpha activity of less than 3-s duration into quiet sleep or indeterminate sleep at a rate greater than one burst per 10 s is not scored as an EEG arousal. Three seconds of alpha sleep is not scored as an arousal unless a 10-s episode of alpha-free sleep precedes it

- Transitions from one sleep state to another are not sufficient of themselves to be scored as EEG arousals unless they meet the criteria indicated above

- Fast activity associated with the high-voltage bursts in EEG with tracé alternant patterns are not considered to be arousals (Figure 4.42)

Arousal classification categories

- *Spontaneous arousal* No discernible precipitating stimulus associated with the arousal (Figure 4.34)

- *Intervention arousal* Obvious observed cause is noted and indicated by annotations of caretaker or technician intervention preceding the arousal (Figure 4.43)

- *Pre-apnea/hypopnea arousal* An arousal that begins within 10 s before the beginning of an apnea. The apnea/hypopnea must be >4 s duration (Figure 4.44). Although the following two respiratory-related arousal types are listed here, criteria are further described in the cardiorespiratory sections

- *Post-apnea/hypopnea arousal* An arousal that begins during or immediately after an apnea/hypopnea. The apnea/hypopnea must be >4 s duration (Figure 4.45)

Classification of arousals with sleep state

The following rules can be used for relating each arousal with a sleep state:

(1) An arousal that occurs within the first half of an epoch is associated with the sleep state of the previous epoch, while an arousal that occurs within the second half of an epoch is associated with the sleep state of the epoch in which the arousal occurs;

(2) Sometimes an arousal leading to wake state occurs within the first epoch of a wake period. In this case the previous epoch of sleep is associated with the arousal.

After arousals are identified, arousal indexes can be calculated for the number of arousals per hour of quiet, active, indeterminate sleep, and total sleep time. A minimum amount of sleep, such as 1 h, should be specified for reporting an arousal index.

CARDIORESPIRATORY EVENTS

IPSG has an important role in the diagnosis of clinically important abnormalities in cardio-respiratory function. The role of the IPSG in the assessment of risk for sudden infant death syndrome in the absence of other high-risk factors remains unresolved.

Cardiorespiratory events and oxygen saturation are of particular interest in infant sleep recordings and their significance may vary with the infant's age. Reliable recognition of cardiorespiratory events and patterns is essential. Typically, the definition of cardiorespiratory events in infants does not differ substantially from scoring in older children. However, there are additional considerations described in the following paragraphs and illustrated primarily with examples from the CHIME study.

Cardiac definitions and arrhythmias

The ECG is an important component of the IPSG. Careful review of the ECG, with particular attention to abnormalities that place the infant at risk for arrhythmias, is important for any infant who has had an apparent life-threatening episode[54]. Sinus bradycardia is commonly seen in association with apneas or vagal stimulation, such as during feeding. As in adult PSGs, the IPSG typically uses a single ECG derivation (lead) that precludes an in-depth analysis of heart structure or disease but permits observation of certain dysrhythmias. A brief description of ECG basics, normal heart rate ranges and abnormal complexes is included here. The reader is referred to general ECG texts such as Davis[55] and Dubin[56] for more detailed information.

The QRS and computation of heart rate

As described in Chapter 3, the ECG in IPSGs may be recorded from modified Lead 1 or modified Lead 2 placements (Figure 3.2). These derivations will show waves of sufficient amplitude so that the entire PQRST complex can be identified. Typical IPSG recording speeds (30-s epochs or 10 mm/s) are not the same as the standard speed used for ECG, 25 mm/s. Because of the slow paper speed and single lead, many of the measurements made by cardiologists can only be approximated in the IPSG. Nevertheless, the normal PQRST complex (Figure 3.17), can be observed and deviations from the norm can be identified. The sleep laboratory must have guidelines in place to specify which deviations should be designated for clinical review or for emergency action (see Table 3.5 for CHIME criteria).

Typical QRS recordings (Figure 4.46) may be distorted by variations in electrode placement, body movement or holding the infant; therefore, documentation of these factors is very important. Polarity of the complex can be accidentally reversed so that the waves appear to be upside down (Figure 3.18). Examples of definite or probable artifacts are shown in Figure 4.47. These artifacts are often eliminated by reversing the leads in the input device or in the leads selected for display. One ECG recording problem that can influence subsequent heart rate computations is a very-low-amplitude R-wave (Figure 4.47a). In this case, computerized systems will not always be able to recognize the R-wave and this situation can result in a false calculation of bradycardia. Conversely, the T-wave amplitude can be as high as that of the R-wave, causing the heart rate to be doubled erroneously. Body movement may produce artifact simulating a

QRS as shown in Figure 4.47b. Movement from respiration also can result in shifting of the ECG baseline and confound the automated computation of heart rate as shown in Figure 4.47c (the abdominal tracing, ABD, shows the respiratory effort). Careful attention must be paid to these situations so that false data are not reported. Criteria for eliminating artifactual cardiac signals are shown in Appendix G.

The basic heart rhythm is called the sinus rhythm[57] because it originates in the sinoatrial (SA) node of the heart. Normally, the intervals between like components of the ECG complex are relatively constant in the calm infant breathing comfortably. However, the heart rate and the intervals between similar components of the ECG vary with activity and vary with respiration. Respiration-related variability in heart rate is called respiratory sinus arrhythmia (RSA). The R–R and P–P intervals shorten during inspiration and lengthen during expiration because changes in the intrathoracic pressure alter cardiac filling and emptying, and thus change blood pressure. In the spontaneously breathing infant, inspiration decreases the blood pressure, thereby reducing stretch of the baroreceptors and causing acceleration of the sinus rate; in contrast, sinus rate is decreased during expiration because baroreceptors are stretched. Any factors that accentuate the changes in pleural pressure during respiration, e.g. airway obstruction, can also accentuate the normal variation in heart rate between inspiration and expiration.

Computation of heart rate

Conventional cardiology techniques for measuring heart rate do not generally apply to PSG recordings due to the different 'chart speed' of the recordings. Laboratories should have a standard method to calculate number of R-waves/min as the heart rate. Rates are expressed as beats per min or bpm. A good heart rate ruler can be calibrated to conform to PSG chart speeds. Computer-assisted acquisition systems typically compute heart rate for you based on the R–R interval.

Normal heart rate ranges for newborns and young infants

Normal heart rate ranges have been established for infants[58] (Table 4.4). These ranges can provide useful references for determining bradycardia and

Table 4.4 Normal electrocardiogram standards for children up to 1 year old. All values given are 2nd and 98th percentiles with mean in parentheses. Adapted from reference 57

	Age						
	0–1 days	1–3 days	3–7 days	7–30 days	1–3 months	3–6 months	6–12 months
Heart rate (beats/min)	94–155 (122)	91–158 (122)	90–166 (128)	106–182 (149)	120–179 (149)	105–185 (141)	108–169 (131)
PR interval, lead II (s)	0.08–0.16 (0.107)	0.08–0.14 (0.108)	0.07–0.15 (0.102)	0.07–0.14 (0.100)	0.07–0.13 (0.098)	0.07–0.15 (0.105)	0.07–0.16 (0.106)
QRS duration, V_5 (s)	0.02–0.07 (0.05)	0.02–0.07 (0.05)	0.02–0.07 (0.05)	0.02–0.08 (0.05)	0.02–0.08 (0.05)	0.02–0.08 (0.05)	0.03–0.08 (0.05)

V_5, axillary line lead placement

tachycardia since the lower and upper heart rate limits change with age.

Traditional polygraph systems can be configured with cardiotachometers to compute heart rate; computerized systems have various techniques for computing and displaying heart rate. Heart rate variability, or lack of variability, also may be of interest in assessing infant status[59]. There have been numerous approaches to quantify heart rate variability and all remain research tools at present.

Arrhythmia

Heart rate values outside the accepted ranges may be of clinical significance and need to be evaluated. Similarly, alterations in conduction should be assessed. In both cases, a complete ECG with limb and precordial leads is useful because rhythm disturbances may be difficult to detect in one lead and readily apparent in another. Furthermore, because of the recent heightened interest about the relationship between long QT and SIDS[60] there is merit in evaluating the ECG of every infant who has polysomnography. Abnormalities of cardiac conduction or rate are referred to as a dysrhythmia or arrhythmia. There are a limited number of arrhythmias that are seen often in the very young infant. Sinus bradycardia is by far the most common (Figure 4.48a). Junctional escape beats (Figure 4.48b), as a function of sinus arrhythmia are also very common. These occur when the sinus rate slows so much that the atrioventricular junction transiently becomes the fastest pacemaker in the

heart and it causes the ventricles to beat (shown by arrows); thus, the junctional tissue has 'escaped' from the suppression of the SA node, which usually beats faster than the junctional tissue. Other arrhythmias that occur less frequently are premature ventricular contractions (PVCs; Figure 4.48c), where the beat is initiated in the ventricle and conduction initially spread through ventricular tissue, which is usually slower than spread through the specialized conduction pathways; this produces a beat that starts with an abnormally wide QRS and has a grossly abnormal complex that occurs earlier than the next expected beat; that is, it is premature. Premature atrial contractions (PACs; Figure 4.48d), appear much like typical SA beats but the complex occurs earlier than expected; sometimes, the P-wave will have a different conformation than the normal beat because the impulse arises in a part of the atrium distant from the SA node. Rarely seen is atrioventricular block (A–V block) produced by aberrant conduction between the atrium and ventricles; this causes either a prolonged P–R interval (1° A–V block) or a failure for the sinus beat to conduct to the ventricle (2° or 3° A–V block), that is, P without QRS. If some P-waves are not conducted but there is a fixed pattern or relationship between the atrial and the ventricular beats that are conducted, this is known as 2° A–V block; if there is no relationship between the atrial and ventricular beats (disassociation), this is 3° A–V block. Another arrhythmia that occurs in infants is paroxysmal atrial tachycardia (PAT; Figure 4.48e), that is, a rapid atrial impulse that can cause conduction through the normal pathways to the ventricle. Because of the very rapid rate, there might also be abnormal conduction to the ventricle causing the complexes to appear abnormal. As mentioned above, there has been an association between long QT (Figure 4.48f) and SIDS. Although it is often difficult to obtain a precise QT interval corrected for heart rate, from a single ECG lead, finding a potentially long QT merits further evaluation by complete ECG.

During an IPSG, all arrhythmias should be documented and brought to the attention of clinical staff. Second and 3° A–V blocks are always pathological and require prompt attention. PAT is pathological, although it may be well tolerated for periods of time; this too requires prompt attention. Both PVCs and PACs are common, although they rarely cause any hemodynamic compromise. Rather, they can represent serious cardiac disease when they are frequent or arise from multiple foci. On the other hand, respiratory sinus arrhythmia with or without junctional escape beats is generally benign. More importantly, when there is very wide variation in the sinus rate, it may indicate the presence of factors that cause large changes in blood pressure, such as airway obstruction. Protocols should be in place regarding urgent notification of clinical personnel and should describe when immediate intervention is required. Since infants may have bradycardia or asystole (Figure 4.48g) that rapidly evolves into respiratory arrest, the ability of staff to apply the criteria for cardiac arrhythmia identification must be regularly evaluated and tested.

A variety of conditions can create unusual QRS complexes that may or may not be artifactual. The rule of thumb is to report any unusual QRS complex.

Respiratory events and patterns

Apnea has been defined as the 'absence of breath', or 'the complete cessation of breathing for more than 10 s in adults and 3 s in infants'[59]. In IPSG recordings, apnea often includes variations such as a reduction of respiratory airflow and/or respiratory effort[61,62]. For example, some computerized systems have filters that search for airflow signals less than some set value such as < 25% of baseline amplitude and will categorize these as apneic rather than hypopneic events. Addition of CO_2 to the airflow measure can help reinforce or supplement thermistor results. In addition, the numerical CO_2

output should be available so that the effects of respiratory insufficiency on CO_2 values can be evaluated and abnormal increases identified. A method for eliminating spurious CO_2 data is given in Appendix G. Each sleep laboratory must set its own amplitude criteria for the definition of apnea. During the IPSG a variety of respiratory disturbances and events can be expected to occur. Indeed, in infants, the signs of respiratory compromise may be more subtle and not as easy to measure as those seen in older children and adults. Infants have all the types of apnea seen in adults, but interpretation of the significance may differ.

Types of apnea

Central apnea

Central apnea is defined as the simultaneous cessation of airflow and effort[7,62] (Figure 4.49). The duration of an apnea consists of the time spent not breathing, that is, from the end of one inspiration to the start of the next inspiration. However, for convenience, it is often measured from the peak of one breath to the peak of the next breath. Although sleep specialists typically define central apnea as a cessation in airflow and effort of ≥ 10 s duration, many pediatric specialists consider any respiratory disturbance to be notable. For example, central apneas can be categorized by durations of < 3 s, 3–6 s, 7–10 s, 11–16 s, 17–20 s and > 20 s or similar categories. The clinical significance of these events is unknown since a central apnea often follows a normal sigh. Some polysomnographers do not consider events following a sigh.

Home apnea monitors are generally set to alarm when apnea monitored by effort sensors or bands exceeds 20-s duration, although shorter events may be recorded without an alarm[63]. Central apnea is the apnea type typically associated with apnea of prematurity and it may be treated with respiratory stimulants[64] and/or discharge from the hospital with a home apnea monitor[65]. The frequency of these events is expected to diminish as the infant matures. Brief central apneas often follow body movements (Figures 4.50 and 4.51) or sighs.

Although this definition seems very clear-cut, in practice, measuring central apnea is not always so straightforward. The CHIME study developed a set of decision points to aid in apnea measurement. These guidelines are given in Appendix F.

Obstructive sleep apnea

Obstructive sleep apnea (OSA) is defined by continued respiratory efforts in the absence of airflow[7,66] (Figure 4.52). Arousals, cardiac dysrhythmias or arrhythmias, and oxygen desaturation are often associated with OSA, but only desaturation and possibly bradycardia are regularly seen in infants. OSA is generally not anticipated in normal infants in the absence of other disease or presence of congestion[67]. Estimates of expected OSA frequencies have been proposed for various age groups, for example, < 1/h of sleep after 3 months of age, no OSA > 10-s duration after 3 months of age and no OSA > 15-s duration in infants < 3 months of age[68]. Observation of completely obstructed events may be infrequent. Respiratory efforts (breaths) in OSA often are out-of-phase, that is, the rib cage and abdomen signals occur in opposite directions (i.e. 180° out-of-phase) at the same time or very close to the same time[69]. Recent reviews of clinical practice guidelines and a technical report for the diagnosis and management of childhood OSA syndrome were recently published by the American Academy of Pediatrics[70,71].

Mixed apnea

Many apneic events include both central apnea and obstructed breaths and are referred to as mixed apneas (Figure 4.53). Some obstructed breaths often follow a central apnea, perhaps due to surface tension foray collapsing the pharynx. A central apnea following obstructed breaths may represent the infant tiring. There is no consensus on when to classify an event as mixed, central or obstructive. For example, in the absence of airflow ≥ 10-s duration, it might be determined that both the central and obstructive components must last at least 3 s to qualify as a mixed event. Another method would be to require at least one or two obstructed breaths within an apnea (Figures 4.54 and 4.55). In adult studies, mixed and obstructed apneas are often grouped together for reporting purposes as both include evidence of obstructed breathing. In adults, mixed apnea is almost always a central component followed by the obstructive portion but, in infants, the reverse may also occur.

Types of hypopnea

As opposed to apnea, which presupposes an absence of airflow, hypopnea is defined as a reduction in, but not complete absence of, airflow. The degree of reduction required to determine when a change in respiration can be defined as a hypopneic event has not been uniformly defined. Part of this difficulty stems from the fact that true flow, pneumotachometer, is rarely measured. Most often, the presence of flow is inferred from measures of nasal temperature and can, therefore, be considered semiquantitative at best. Hypopnea can also be central or obstructive in nature. Definitions of hypopnea developed for CHIME IPSG interpretation follow.

Central hypopnea

CHIME defined central hypopnea as a 50% decrease in the amplitude of the thermistor channel lasting 10 s or more with in-phase rib cage and abdominal movements. Since the thermistor is not a readily quantifiable measure of airflow and is subject to considerable artifacts, in order to qualify, one of two additional criteria must be fulfilled: the event must be followed by a drop in oxyhemoglobin saturation (SaO_2) of 4% or more or an arousal confirmed by EEG. An example of a possible central hypopnea of less than 10-s duration is shown in Figure 4.56.

Obstructive hypopnea (partial obstruction)

As compared to central hypopnea, obstructive hypopnea was defined as a 50% decrease in the amplitude of the thermistor signal lasting 10 s or more with rib cage and abdominal movement partially or completely out-of-phase. Since the thermistor is not a readily quantifiable measure of airflow and is subject to considerable artifacts, in order to qualify, one of two additional criteria must be fulfilled: the event must be accompanied by a drop in SaO_2 of 4% or more, or an arousal confirmed on EEG (Figure 4.57). An illustration of the differences between central and obstructive hypopnea is given in Figure 4.58.

Breathing patterns

Periodic breathing

Periodic breathing (PB) is a pattern of repetitive central apneas[72,73]. One definition of PB[74] is the presence of three or more central apneas of > 3-s duration each, separated by three to four normal breaths or less than 20 s of breathing (Figure 4.59). PB is common in normal infants and its clinical importance is debated. PB can be associated with oxygen desaturation on a transient, event-related basis or in a progressive, chronic pattern[75]. The clinical relevance of PB is not clear. It may result from the instability of the cardiorespiratory system, similar to Cheyne-Stokes breathing in adults.

Paradoxical breathing

Paradoxical breathing (PDB) is a common finding in infants, particularly during AS or REM sleep. PDB is defined by out-of-phase breaths in the rib cage and abdominal respiratory effort tracings (Figure 4.60). Inductance plethysmography is particularly useful for displaying this pattern. It has been suggested that PDB may be indicative of obstructed breathing even though IPSGs often reveal little or no change in airflow amplitudes during these periods. When OSA is present, the rib cage and abdominal respiratory effort channels can often be seen to change from synchronous in-phase breathing prior to the event and evolve into out-of-phase breaths during the event. If effort is being monitored with piezo bands, observation of the infant is required to verify out-of-phase breathing since band displacement can present as out-of-phase breaths. As with PB, PDB can be accompanied by oxygen desaturation.

CHIME's detailed procedures for measuring apnea

Refinements in the methods typically used in measuring respiratory events were developed in the CHIME study[63,69]. These definitions and procedures are described here in order to provide the reader with a set of tools that may prove useful. During the CHIME research study the IPSG recordings of respiratory effort were obtained from the respiratory inductance plethysmography (RIP) sensors of the CHIME monitor and recorded in parallel on the monitor and the IPSG recording. The first set of apnea definitions involves airflow (CO_2 and thermistor). The initial step is to determine the baseline amplitudes for breaths prior to the potential event.

The criteria applied are:

(1) It precedes the event;

(2) Contains at least three deflections;

(3) Does not contain sighs or obvious artifacts;

(4) It is the closest activity to the potential event that meets these criteria.

Using a computerized recording system, placement of cursors at the base and top of these deflections will yield the average amplitudes. Second, apnea duration is measured. In the thermistor channel, mark the peaks of the two deflections that represent the largest interval between deflections that are $\geq 25\%$ of the baseline for this channel. For CO_2, mark the initial increase in CO_2 of the two deflections that represent the longest interval between deflections that are $\geq 75\%$ of the baseline amplitude for CO_2. If the duration exceeds the criterion for an apnea, record this as an apnea. Third, if there are no deflections in the RIP SUM, RC and ABD channels then this apnea is a central event. To determine whether the event is an obstructed apnea, CHIME identified and counted the number of out-of-phase breaths that occurred within the interval measured in step 2 above (see Figure 4.55). Out-of-phase deflections were defined as ABD and RC signals that occurred in opposite directions (180 degrees out-of-phase) at the same or very close to the same time. If RIP is not available, the presence of breaths recorded from the RC and/or ABD in the absence of airflow (meeting the no airflow criteria) are considered to be obstructed or mixed apneas as described in the earlier sections.

Oxygen saturation

Baseline oxygen saturation levels in infants are expected to remain within a relatively limited range (100% to 96%)[75-77]. Factors that can affect the oximeter reading include movement, poor contact of the sensor that allows ambient light to be detected, or a very cold or warm extremity that may affect the peripheral circulation. Condition of the sensor should be examined when opportunities arise during feeding or other interventions.

To validate the SaO_2 percentage values that are the usual output recorded during an IPSG, the pulse waveform should be added to the montage. Observation of the degradation of the pulse waveform will identify periods where the SaO_2 percentage is partially, or completely, unreliable (see Figure 4.53). Transient periods of desaturation may accompany apneic events (see Figure 4.50).

Recovery to baseline within seconds should be anticipated. Some infants may present a relatively low SaO_2 baseline, and therefore, desaturation during an event will be more pronounced due to the shape of the oxyhemoglobin dissociation curve. The clinical protocol should address the appropriate action to take for desaturation. In order to make correct determinations of SaO_2, it is necessary to record the pulse waveform so that low values due to poor pulse signal and movement artifacts do not result in inappropriate interventions. A method for eliminating spurious saturation values from scoring results is given in Appendix G. In some cases where baseline values are lower than expected, it may be prudent to assess the infant's temperature and the ambient temperature and make adjustments as indicated.

IPSG REPORTS

Polysomnogram recordings have two primary goals: first, to outline a detailed array of parameters related to sleep architecture, and second, to identify events involving other recorded neurobiological parameters, such as cardiorespiratory and motility responses throughout the course of sleep. Customarily these details are summarized in a PSG report (Figure 4.61), accompanied by a sleep hypnogram (Figure 4.62). An abstracted outline of the categories or sections usually included in this PSG report along with illustrative and explanatory comments relative to each of these broad categories are as reviewed below.

Sleep summary

Amount of time for describing sleep parameters is dependent on the total period beginning with 'Lights out' and ending at 'Lights on'. This interval constitutes the reference for calculating measures such as time in bed, latency to sleep and wake time before and during sleep. The total time, percent and latency for the various state and stage categories can be determined and included here.

Respiratory summary

The designation 'cardiorespiratory', is comprised of respiratory, cardiac and oxygen saturation results. Central, obstructive and mixed apnea along with

hypopneic episodes are tallied and totals are listed in terms of the sleep state or stage at the time of occurrence along with average duration (in seconds). An Apnea Index (AI) and an Apnea plus Hypopnea Index (AHI) can be calculated as the number of apnea or apnea plus hypopnea events divided by the total sleep time multiplied by 60. No specific normal threshold for infants has been universally established.

Oxygen saturation summary

SaO_2 percent values are presented in relation to sleep states and stages or in relation to apnea/hypopnea events. A critical level or levels can be defined, for example, as time below 96% or 91%, according to sleep laboratory criteria.

Cardiac summary

The ECG is evaluated in terms of heart rate averages and ranges relative to sleep state or stage and wake conditions. In addition, cardiac arrythmias are noted and related to time of occurrence, appearance and association with respiratory events or other stimuli such as feedings.

Bodily activity summary

While the report suggests a brief overall picture of movement time, it is clear that an index can be derived which will supply a more meaningful diagnostic impression. Overall, PSG results can be summarized in a 'comments' section and the report customarily concludes with statements detailing clinical diagnostic impressions.

Sleep hypnogram

Another strategy for providing a general picture of the sleep study is a description in terms of a hypnogram or somnogram. Although illustrated earlier in the material on smoothing (Figure 4.34), here the emphasis is on the graphical outlining of the sequence of sleep states or stages across the night. Figure 4.62 is a simplified portrayal of smoothed sleep states, clearly showing the possibilities for a graphic representation of the interactions between sleep state parameters. As can be quickly seen the hypnogram has the possibility for a visual depiction of developing ultradian cycling.

Computer-assisted analysis

Polysomnogram scoring details presented here have relied on visual and manual, although at times computer-assisted, analysis techniques. This perspective reflects not only current assessment strategies, but highlights the increasing adoption of computerized sleep data acquisition and scoring techniques. Guidelines, as described by Hirshkowitz and Moore[78], are needed to resolve issues revolving around recording, scoring, monitoring and statistical evaluation standards. Although, as of now, the attempts to introduce a so-called paperless polysomnogram have been limited, the present status most relevant to IPSG does reveal a variety of productive efforts pertaining to infant sleep analyses. The system of Scher and colleagues[79] emerges most prominently as one example of the feasibility of computer signal processing and analysis to study the ontogeny of sleep. Other potential analytic approaches for differentiating EEG signals relative to sleep epochs are spectral analysis[80], wavelet transforms[81], tree-based neural network system[82] and zero-crossing measures[83]. Although all of these may be employed, automated results still require reliability comparison with manually scored results. The work scope is challenging.

SUMMARY

While the prime purpose of the IPSG is rooted in a description of the current neurophysiological functional sleep states of an infant, several other equally important results of the process need to be emphasized. First, there is always an inherent data lode that can be mined for research. These possibilities may vary from a purely maturational description of developmental sleep states/stages to a detailed examination of the co-variations of specific sleep parameters related to induced or endogenous stimuli. *A propos* the developmental perspective, the collection of cross-sectional and longitudinal data focused on specific central or autonomic nervous system variables provide the basic data for observations on the ontogeny of sleep organization. Although challenging, the IPSG has just begun to reveal facets of the complex ontogeny of sleep and its potential for research and clinical assessment.

REFERENCES

1. Curzi-Dascalova L, Monod N, Guidasci S, *et al.* Transition veille-sommeil chez les nouveau-nés et les nourrisson avant l'âge de 3 mois. *Rev EEG Neurophysiol* 1981;11:1–10

2. Dreyfus-Brisac C. Neonatal electroencephalography. In Scarpelli EM, Cosmi EV, eds. *Review of Perinatal Medicine*, Vol. 3. New York: Raven Press, 1979:397–472

3. Dreyfus-Brisac C. Ontogenesis of brain bioelectrical activity and sleep organization in neonates and infants. In Falkner F, Tanner JM, eds. *Human Growth*, Vol. 3. New York: Plenum Publishing Corporation, 1979:157–82

4. Lindsley DB. A longitudinal study of the occipital alpha rhythm in normal children: frequency and amplitude standards. *J Gen Psychol* 1939;55:197–213

5. Niedermeyer E. Maturation of the EEG: development of waking and sleep patterns. In Niedermeyer E, Lopes da Silva F, eds. *Electroencephalography: Basic Principles, Clinical Applications, and Related Fields*, 4th edn. Philadelphia: Lippincott, Williams & Wilkins, 1999:189–214

6. Anders T, Emde RL, Parmelee A, eds. *A Manual of Standardized Terminology, Techniques and Criteria for Scoring of States of Sleep and Wakefulness in Newborn Infants*. Los Angeles, CA: UCLA Brain Information Service/BRS Publications Office, 1971

7. Brouillette RT. Assessing cardiopulmonary function during sleep in infants and children. In Beckerman RC, Brouillette RT, Hunt CE, eds. *Respiratory Control Disorders in Infants and Children*. Baltimore: Williams & Wilkins, 1992:125–41

8. Guilleminault C, Souquet M. Sleep states and related pathology. In Korobkin R, Guilleminault C, eds. *Advances in Perinatal Neurology*. New York: Spectrum Publications, 1979:225–47

9. Haddad GG, Jung HJ, Lai TJ, *et al.* Determination of sleep state in infants using respiratory variability. *Pediatr Res* 1987;21:556–62

10. Hoppenbrouwers T, Ruiz ME, Geidel S, *et al.* Electronic monitoring in the newborn infant: technical guidelines. In Guilleminault C, ed. *Sleep and Waking Disorders: Indications and Techniques.* Menlo Park, CA: Addison-Wesley, 1982:61–98

11. Curzi-Dascalova L, Mirmiran M. *Manual of Methods for Recording and Analyzing Sleep-Wakefulness States in Pre-term and Full-Term Infants.* Paris: Les Editions INSERM, 1996

12. Crowell DH, Kapuniai LE, Boychuk RB, *et al.* Daytime sleep stage organization in three-month-old infants. *Electroencephalogr Clin Neurophysiol* 1982;53:36–47

13. Rechtschaffen A, Kales A, eds. *A Manual of Standardized Terminology, Techniques and Scoring System for Sleep Stages of Human Subjects.* National Institutes of Health Publication No. 204. Washington DC: US Government Printing Office, 1968

14. Hughes JR. Development of sleep spindles in the first year of life. *J Clin Neurophysiol* 1996;27:107–15

15. Sheldon SH, Riter S, Detrojan M. *Atlas of Sleep Medicine in Infants and Children.* Armonk, NY: Futura Publishing, 1999

16. Stockard-Pope JE, Werner SS, Bickford RG. *Atlas of Neonatal Electroencephalography*, 2nd edn. New York: Raven Press, 1992

17. Kooi, KA, Taucker RP, Marshall RE. *Fundamentals of Electroencephalography*, 2nd edn. New York: Harper & Row, 1978

18. Metcalf D, Mondale J, Butler F. Ontogenesis of spontaneous K-complexes. *Psychophysiology* 1971;8:340–7

19. Spehlmann R. *EEG Primer.* Amsterdam: Elsevier/North Holland Biomedical Press, 1981

20. Crowell DH, Brooks LJ, Colton R, *et al.* Infant polysomnography: reliability. *Sleep* 1997;20:553–60

21. Aserinsky E, Kleitman N. Regularly occurring periods of eye motility and concomitant phenomena, during sleep. *Science* 1953;118:273–4

22. Dreyfus-Brisac C. Ontogenesis of sleep in early human prematurity from 21–27 weeks of conceptional age. *Dev Psychobiol* 1968;2:162–9

23. Prechtl H, Lenard H. A study of eye movements in sleeping newborn infants. *Brain Res* 1967;5:477–93

24. Dreyfus-Brisac C. Ontogenesis of human sleep in human prematures after 32 weeks of conceptional age. *Dev Psychobiol* 1970;3:91–121

25. Parmelee AH, Stern E. Development of states in infants. In Clemente CD, Purpura DP, Mayer FE, eds. *Sleep and the Maturing Nervous System.* New York: Academic Press, 1972;200–28

26. Liefting B, Bes F, Fagioli I, *et al.* Electromyographic activity and sleep states in infants. *Sleep* 1994;17:718–22

27. Parmelee A. The ontogeny of sleep patterns and associated periodicities in infants. In Falkner F, Kretchmer N, Rossi E, eds. *Modern Problems in Pediatrics. Vol. 2. Prenatal and Postnatal Development of the Human Brain.* Basel: Karger AG, 1974:298–311

28. Peirano P, Curzi-Dascalova L, Korn G. Influence of sleep state and age on body motility in normal premature and full-term neonates. *Neuropediatrics* 1986;17:186–90

29. Peirano P, Curzi-Dascalova L. Modulation of motor activity patterns and sleep states in low-risk prematurely born infants reaching normal term: a comparison with full-term newborns. *Neuropediatrics* 1995;26:8–13

30. Anders, T. The infant sleep profile. *Neuropediatrics* 1974;5:425–42

31. Kulp TD, Corwin MJ, Brooks LJ, *et al.* The effect of epoch length and smoothing on infant sleep and waking state architecture in term infants at 42–46 weeks postconceptional age. *Sleep* 2000;23:893–9

32. Guilleminault C, Souquet M. Appendix II. *Sleep and Waking Disorders: Indications and Techniques.* Menlo Park, CA: Addison-Wesley Publishing, 1982:415–26

33. Ellingson RJ, Peters JF. Development of EEG and daytime sleep patterns in normal full-term infants during the first 3 months of life: longitudinal observations. *Electroencephalogr Clin Neurophysiol* 1980; 49:112–24

34. Ellingson RJ, Peters JF. Development of EEG and daytime sleep patterns in low risk premature infants during the first year of life: longitudinal observations. *Electroencephalogr Clin Neurophysiol* 1980;50:165–71

35. Harper RM, Leake B, Miyahara L, *et al.* Temporal sequencing in sleep and waking states during the first 6 months of life. *Ex Neurol* 1981;72:294–307

36. Anders TF, Sadeh A, Appareddy V. Normal sleep in neonates and children. In Ferber R, Kryger M, eds. *Principles and Practice of Sleep Medicine in the Child.* Philadelphia: W.B. Saunders, 1992:7–18

37. Emde RN, Walker S. Longitudinal study of infant sleep: results of 14 subjects studied at monthly intervals. *Psychophysiology* 1976;13:456–61

38. Phillipson EA, Sullivan CE. Arousal: the forgotten response to respiratory stimuli. *Am Rev Resp Dis* 1978;118:807–9

39. Scher MS, Steppe DA, Dahl RE, *et al.* Comparison of EEG sleep measures in healthy full-term and preterm infants at matched conceptional ages. *Sleep* 1992;15:442–8

40. Steriade M. Arousal: revisiting the reticular activating system. *Science* 1996;272:225–6

41. Rainnie DG, Grunze HCR, McCarley RW, *et al.* Adenosine inhibition of mesopontine cholinergic neurons: implications for EEG arousal. *Science* 1994;261:689–92

42. Berry RB, Gleeson K. Respiratory arousal from sleep: mechanism and significance. *Sleep* 1997;20:654–75

43. Coons S, Guilleminault C. Motility and arousal in near miss sudden infant death syndrome. *J Pediatr* 1985;107:728–32

44. Hunt CE. Impaired arousal from sleep: relationship to sudden infant death syndrome. *J Perinatol* 1989;9:184–7

45. McNamara F, Issa FG, Sullivan CE. Arousal pattern following central and obstructive breathing abnormalities in infants and children. *J Appl Physiol* 1996;81:2651–7

46. McNamara F, Wulbrand H, Thach BT. Characteristics of the infant arousal response. *J Appl Physiol* 1998;85:2314–21

47. Mograss MA, Ducharme FM, Brouillette RT. Movement/arousals: description, classification and relationship to sleep apnea in children. *Am J Res Crit Care Med* 1994;150:1690–6

48. Mosko S, Richard C, McKenna J. Infant arousals during mother-infant bed sharing: implications for infant sleep and Sudden Infant Death Syndrome research. *Pediatrics* 1997;1200:841–9

49. Thoppil CK, Belan MA, Cowen CP, *et al.* Behavioral arousal in newborn infants and its association with termination of apnea. *J Appl Physiol* 1991;70:2479–84

50. Coons S, Guilleminault C. Development of sleep–wake patterns and non-rapid eye movement sleep stages during the first six months of life in normal infants. *Pediatrics* 1982;69:793–8

51. Crowell DH, Kulp TD, Kapuniai LE, *et al.* Infant polysomnography: reliability and validity of infant arousal assessment. *J Clin Neurophysiol* 2002;19:469–83

52. *Webster's Third International Dictionary*. Springfield, MA: G. & C. Merriam Company, 1961

53. Atlas Task Force. EEG arousals: scoring rules and examples. A preliminary report from the sleep disorders Atlas Task Force of the American Sleep Disorders Association. *Sleep* 1992;15:174–84

54. Pincus SM, Cummins TR, Haddad GG. Heart rate control in normal and aborted-SIDS infants. *Am J Physiol* 1993;264:R638–40

55. Davis D. *Differential Diagnosis of Arrhythmias*. Philadelphia: WB Saunders Company, 1992

56. Dubin D. *Rapid Interpretation of EKGs*, 5th edn. Tampa, FL: Cover, Inc., 1996

57. Pikkujamsa SM, Makikallio TH, Sourander LB, *et al.* Cardiac interbeat interval dynamics from childhood to senescence: comparison of conventional and new measures based on fractals and chaos theory. *Circulation* 1999;100:393–9

58. Van Hare GF, Dubin AM. The normal electrocardiogram. In Allen HD, Clark EB, Gutgesell HP, Driscoll DJ, eds. *Moss and Adams Heart Disease in Infants, Children and Adolescents: Including the Fetus and Young Adult*, 6th edn. Baltimore, MD: Lippincott, Williams & Wilkins 2000:425–42

59. Kryger MH. Monitoring respiratory and cardiac functions. In Kryger MH, Roth T, Dement W, eds. *Principles and Practice of Sleep Medicine*, 3rd edn. Philadelphia: W.B. Saunders, 2000:1217–30

60. Schwartz PJ, Stramba-Badiale M, Segantini A, *et al.* Prolongation of the QT interval and the sudden infant death syndrome. *N Eng J Med* 1998;338:1709–14

61. Ward SL, Marcus CL. Obstructive sleep apnea in infants and young children. *J Clin Neurophysiol* 1996;13:198–207

62. Richards JM, Alexander JR, Shinebourne EA, *et al.* Sequential 22-hour profiles of breathing patterns and heart rate in 110 full-term infants during their first six months of life. *Pediatrics* 1984;74:763–77

63. Ramanathan R, Corwin MJ, Hunt CE, *et al.* Cardiorespiratory events recorded on home monitors: a comparison of healthy infants with those at increased risk for SIDS. *J Am Med Assoc* 2001;285:2199–207

64. Gannon BA. Theophylline or caffeine: which is best for apnea of prematurity? *Neonatal Netw* 2000;19:33–6

65. Perfect Sychowski S, Dodd E, Thomas P, *et al*. Home apnea monitor use in preterm infants discharged from newborn intensive care units. *Pediatrics* 2001;139:245–8

66. Dyson M, Beckerman RC, Brouillette RT. Obstructive sleep apnea syndrome. In Beckerman RC, Brouillette RT, Hunt CE, eds. *Respiratory Control Disorders in Infants and Children.* Baltimore, MD: Williams & Wilkins, 1992:212–30

67. Guilleminault C, Stoohs R. From apnea of infancy to obstructive sleep apnea in the young child. *Chest* 1992;102:1065–71

68. Carroll JL, Loughlin GM. Obstructive sleep apnea syndrome in infants and children: diagnosis and management. In Ferber R, Kryger M, eds. *Principles and Practice of Sleep Medicine in the Child.* Philadelphia: W.B. Saunders, 1995:193–216

69. Weese-Mayer, DE, Corwin MJ, Peucker MR, *et al*. Comparison of apnea identified by respiratory inductance plethysmography with that detected by end-tidal CO_2 or thermistor. The CHIME Study Group. *Am J Respir Crit Care Med* 2000;162:471–80

70. American Academy of Pediatrics. Clinical practice guidelines: diagnostics and management of childhood obstructive sleep apnea syndrome. *Pediatrics* 2002;109:704–12

71. American Academy of Pediatrics. Technical Report: Diagnostics and management of childhood obstructive sleep apnea syndrome. *Pediatrics* 2002;109:1–20

72. Glotzbach SF, Baldwin RB, Lederer BA, *et al*. Periodic breathing in preterm infants: incidence and characteristics. *Pediatrics* 1989;84:785–92

73. Glotzbach SF, Tansey PA, Baldwin RB, *et al*. Periodic breathing parameter values depend on specific pneumogram scoring criteria. *Pediatr Pulmonol* 1989;7:18–21

74. Kelly DH, Shannon D. Periodic breathing in infants with near-miss sudden infant death syndrome. *Pediatrics* 1979;63:355–9

75. Hunt CE, Corwin MJ, Lister G, *et al*. Longitudinal assessment of hemoglobin oxygen saturation in healthy infants during the first 6 months of life. *J Pediatr* 1999;134:580–6

76. Gries RE, Brooks LJ. Normal oxyhemoglobin saturation during sleep. How long does it go? *Chest* 1996;110:1489–92

77. Poets CF, Stebbins VA, Lang JA, *et al*. Arterial oxygen saturation in healthy term infants. *Eur J Pediatr* 1996;155:219–23

78. Hirshkowitz M, Moore CA. Issues in computerized polysomnography. *Sleep* 1994;17:105–12

79. Scher MS, Guthrie RD, Krieger D, *et al*. Maturational aspects of sleep from birth through early childhood. In Beckerman RC, Brouillete RT, Hunt CE, *et al*., eds. *Respiratory Control in Infants and Children.* Baltimore, MD: Williams & Wilkins, 1992: 89–111

80. Litscher G, Pfurtscheller G, Bes F, *et al*. Respiration and heart rate variation in normal infants during quiet sleep in the first year of life. *Klin Pediatr* 1993;205:170–5

81. Jobert M, Tismer C, Poiseau E, *et al*. Wavelets – a new tool in sleep biosignal analysis. *J Sleep Res* 1994;3:223–32

82. Huupponen E, Hasan J, Varri A, *et al*. Arousal detection with a neural network. *J Sleep Res* 1996;5:97

83. Drinnan MJ, Murray A, White JES, *et al*. Automated recognition of EEG changes accompanying arousal in respiratory sleep disorders. *Sleep* 1996;19:296–303

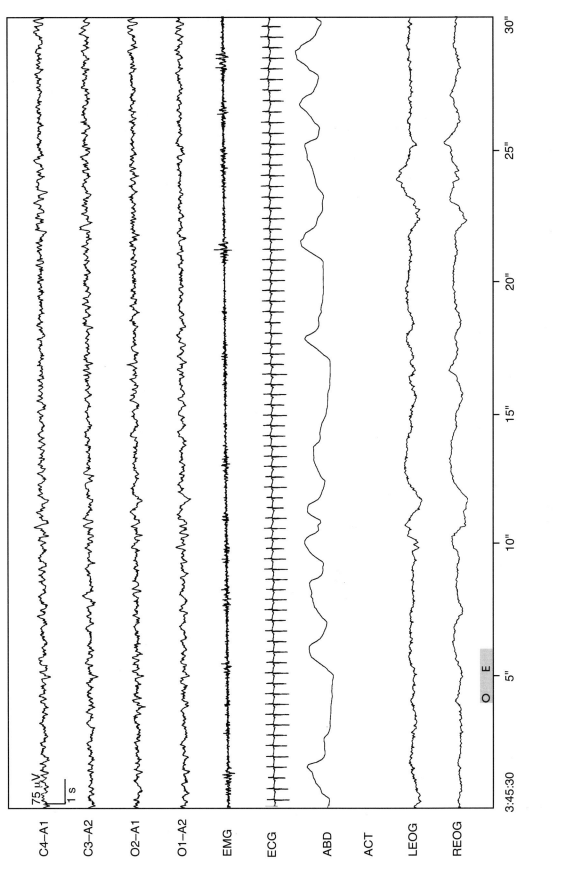

Figure 4.1 Quiet awake beginning at the 'open eyes' (OE) comment in an infant of 39 weeks' gestational age, 45 weeks' conceptional age. Note the low-voltage mixed-frequency electroencephalogram (C4–A1 to O1–A2) and irregular abdominal (ABD) respiration. EMG, submental electromyogram; ECG, electrocardiogram; ACT, actimeter; LEOG, REOG, left and right electrooculogram, respectively

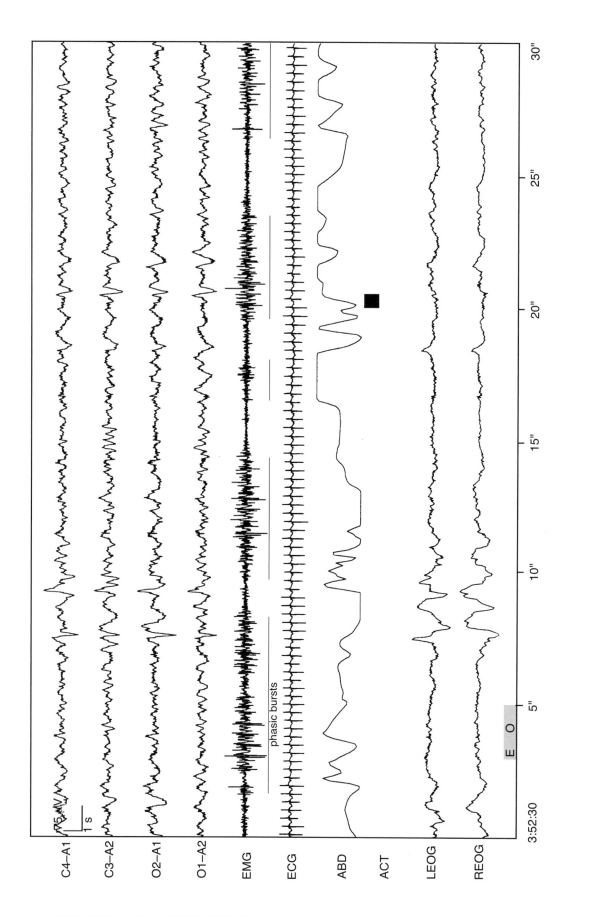

Figure 4.2 Active awake beginning at the 'eyes open' (EO) comment in an infant of 39 weeks' gestational age, 45 weeks' conceptional age. Note the phasic chin electromyogram (EMG) activity (underlined) and rapid eye movements in the left and right electrooculogram (LEOG and REOG) channels. ECG, electrocardiogram; ABD, abdominal respiration; ACT, actimeter

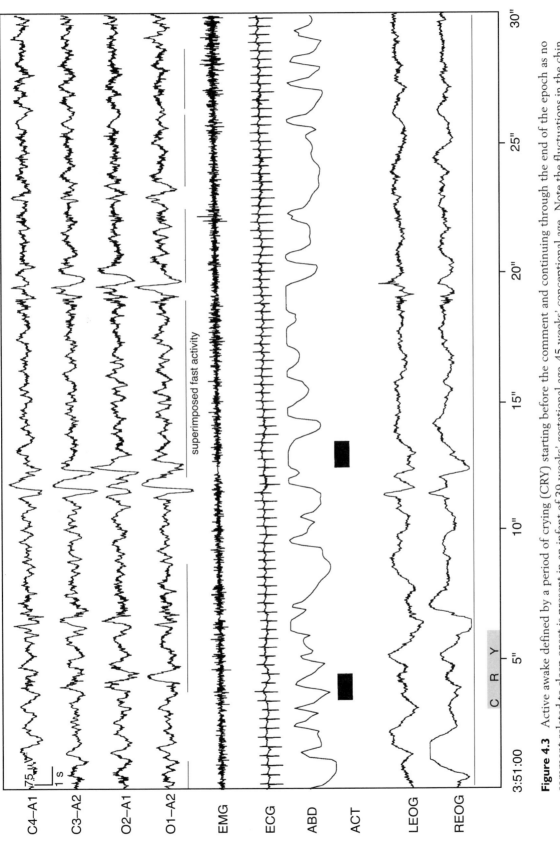

Figure 4.3 Active awake defined by a period of crying (CRY) starting before the comment and continuing through the end of the epoch as no comment related to sleep onset is present in an infant of 39 weeks' gestational age, 45 weeks' conceptional age. Note the fluctuations in the chin electromyogram (EMG), along with the movements (black bars in the actimeter, ACT) and muscle artifacts (fast frequency activity underlined) in the electroencephalogram (C4–A1 to O1–A2) and left and right electrooculogram (LEOG, REOG) (underlined), the very irregular abdominal respirations (ABD) and baseline fluctuations in the electrocardiogram (ECG)

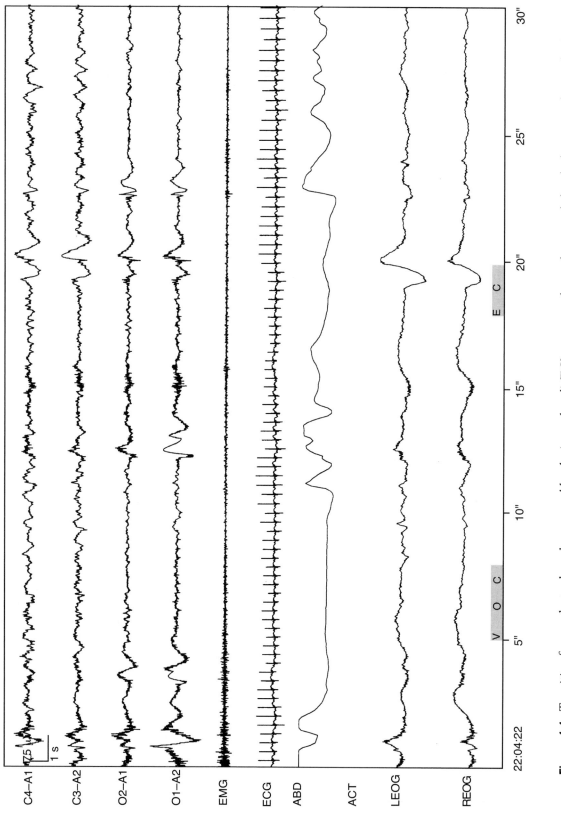
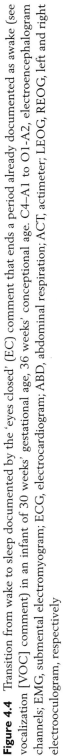

Figure 4.4 Transition from wake to sleep documented by the 'eyes closed' (EC) comment that ends a period already documented as awake (see vocalization [VOC] comment) in an infant of 30 weeks' gestational age, 36 weeks' conceptional age. C4-A1 to O1-A2, electroencephalogram channels; EMG, submental electromyogram; ECG, electrocardiogram; ABD, abdominal respiration; ACT, actimeter; LEOG, REOG, left and right electrooculogram, respectively

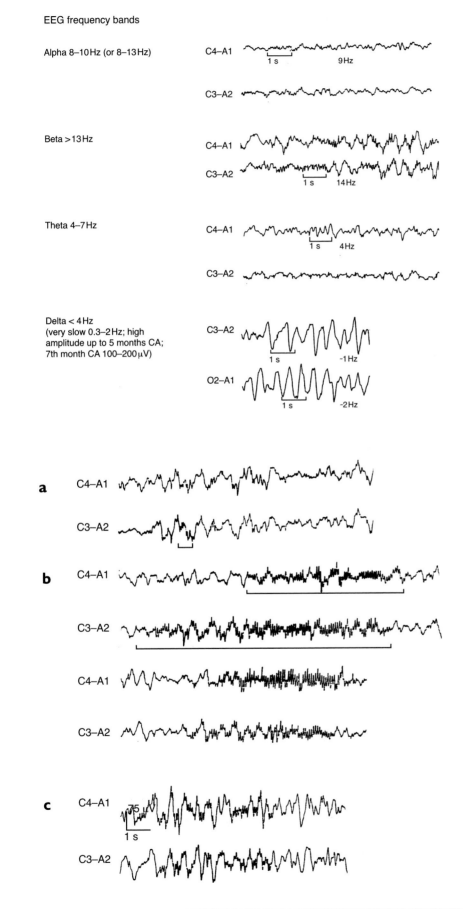

EEG frequency bands

Alpha 8–10Hz (or 8–13Hz)

C4–A1

1 s   9Hz

C3–A2

Beta >13Hz

C4–A1

C3–A2

1 s   14Hz

Theta 4–7Hz

C4–A1

1 s   4Hz

C3–A2

Delta < 4Hz
(very slow 0.3–2Hz; high
amplitude up to 5 months CA;
7th month CA 100–200μV)

C3–A2

1 s   -1Hz

O2–A1

1 s   -2Hz

Figure 4.5
Electroencephalogram (EEG) frequency bands and waveform examples. CA, conceptional age

a   C4–A1

C3–A2

b   C4–A1

C3–A2

C4–A1

C3–A2

c   C4–A1

1 s

C3–A2

Figure 4.6 Sleep spindle development in central electroencephalogram (C4–A1, C3–A2) prior to and after 6 weeks post-term (46 weeks' conceptional age (CA)). a, Evidence of rudimentary or 'pre-spindles' (underlined) that may occur prior to 46 weeks' CA. b, The spindles in C4–A1 are of shorter duration than those in C3–A2 appearing as asynchronous spindles at 46 weeks' CA. c, Spindles are superimposed on delta waves and in a more synchronous fashion at 52 weeks' CA

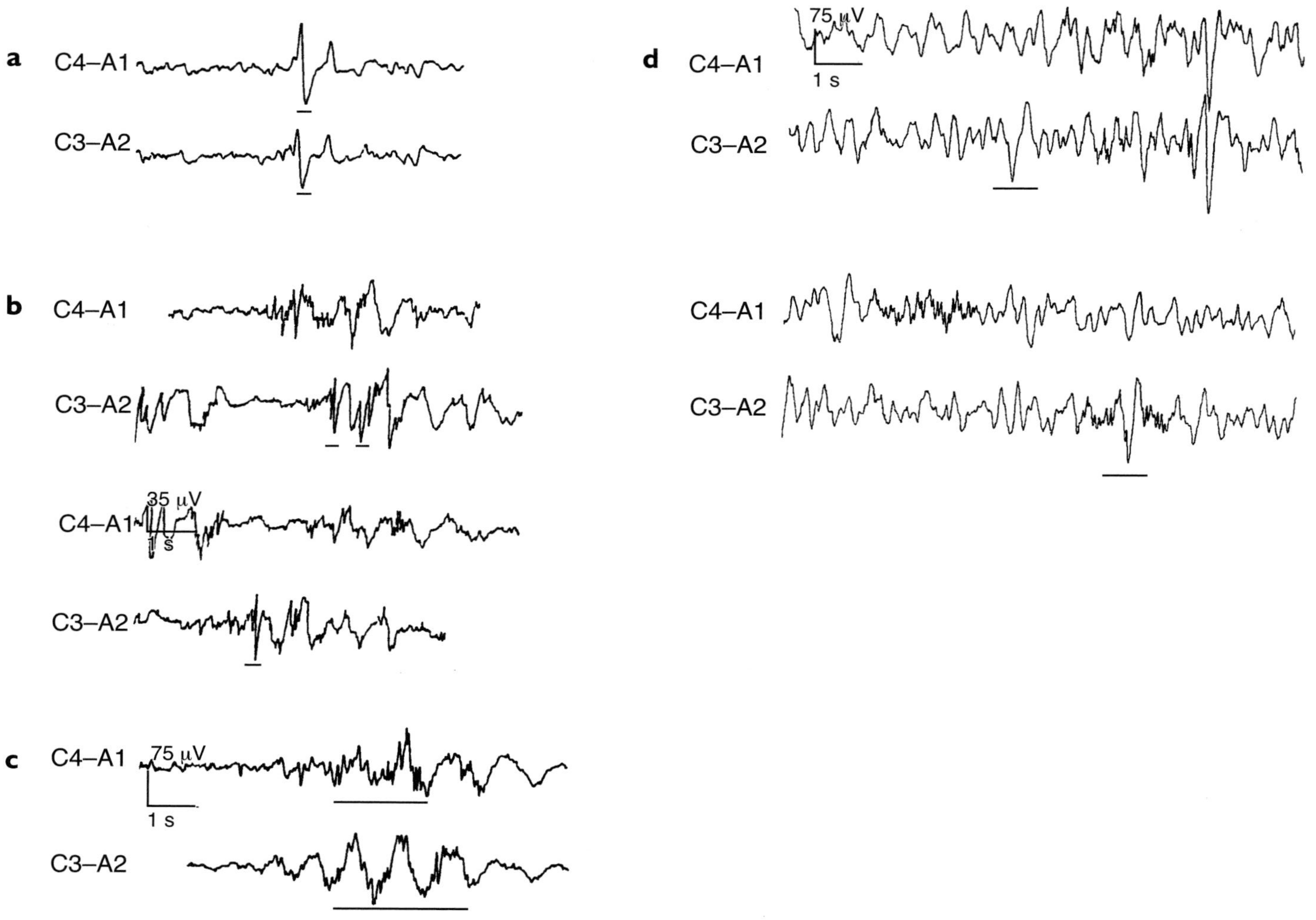

Figure 4.7 Normal features in infant electroencephalogram (EEG) < 6 months adjusted age. a, The sharp transient (underlined) has an initial negative deflection followed by a positive and then another negative wave; b, (underlined) a number of sharp transients precede delta waves. Note the 35 μV scale. c, The delta waves (underlined) have faster frequencies superimposed; this pattern is referred to as delta-brush and is common in premature infants between 32 and 40 weeks' conceptional age. In older infants (6 months adjusted age), K-complexes begin to appear; d, these complexes are recognized by the initial negative wave followed by a positive slow wave that may have spindles superimposed (see underlines)

Conceptional age (weeks)	24	28	32	36	40	44
Awake					Diffuse low voltage	Irregular theta and irregular delta activity
Active sleep Irregular breathing Frequent eye and limb movements No tonic submental EMG				Continuous slow waves 1–2 Hz	Continuous theta, delta	Mixed low voltage irregular, 2–4 Hz slow waves
		a. bursts ≤ 20 s, delta ≥ theta ≥ alpha	1–2 s 4–6 Hz	1–2 Hz		Tracé alternant a. bursts of 4–5 s 1–3 Hz
Quiet sleep Regular breathing No eye and limb movement Tonic submental EMG		b. pauses: no activity ≤ 3 min		shorter pauses	low voltage may appear	b. low voltage activity, 4–5 s Continuous high amplitude slow waves
				Frontal sharp transient and sporadic spikes		
			Delta brushes 10–20 Hz on 0.3–1 Hz			

Chronologic age (months post-term)	2	3	4	5	6
Awake	Irregular low voltage theta				
Active sleep (REM sleep) Irregular breathing Frequent rapid eye movements Low tonic submental EMG	Mixed low voltage irregular, 2–4 Hz slow waves				
Quiet sleep (NREM sleep)	Tracé alternant a. bursts of 4–5 s 1–3 Hz b. low voltage activity, 4–5 s c. High voltage slow waves, 1–2 Hz	Transition to NREM stages of < 20% with spindles = Stage 2; 20–50% = Stage 3; > 50% = Stage 4 Sleep spindles			Incipient K-complexes

Figure 4.8 Maturation of physiological parameters associated with awake and sleep states between 24 weeks' conceptional age and 6 months post-term. Adapted from reference 19. REM, rapid eye movement; EMG, electromyogram

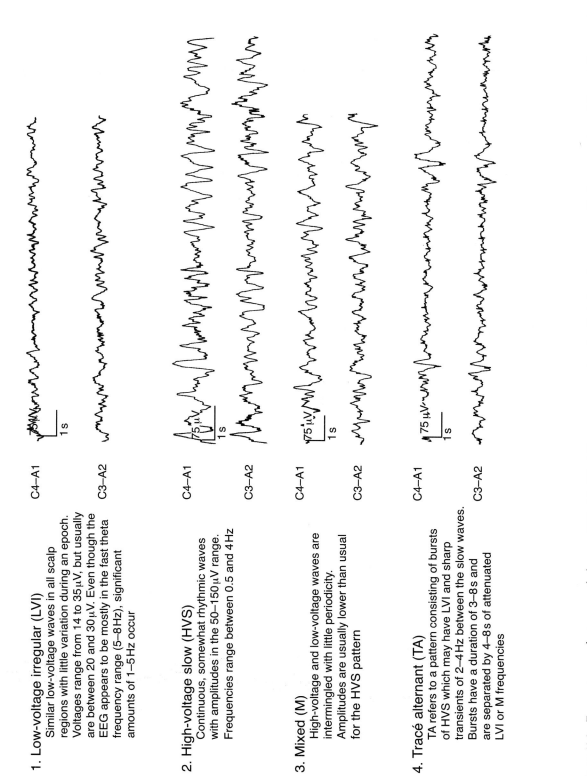

1. Low-voltage irregular (LVI)
Similar low-voltage waves in all scalp regions with little variation during an epoch. Voltages range from 14 to 35 µV, but usually are between 20 and 30 µV. Even though the EEG appears to be mostly in the fast theta frequency range (5–8 Hz), significant amounts of 1–5 Hz occur

2. High-voltage slow (HVS)
Continuous, somewhat rhythmic waves with amplitudes in the 50–150 µV range. Frequencies range between 0.5 and 4 Hz

3. Mixed (M)
High-voltage and low-voltage waves are intermingled with little periodicity. Amplitudes are usually lower than usual for the HVS pattern

4. Tracé alternant (TA)
TA refers to a pattern consisting of bursts of HVS which may have LVI and sharp transients of 2–4 Hz between the slow waves. Bursts have a duration of 3–8 s and are separated by 4–8 s of attenuated LVI or M frequencies

Figure 4.9 Four primary electroencephalogram (C4–A1, C3–A2) patterns associated with infant sleep states. Definitions adapted from reference 6

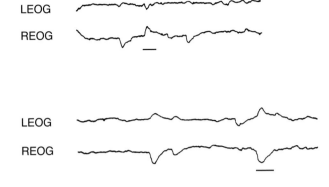

LEOG

REOG

LEOG

REOG

Figure 4.10 Rapid eye movements in left and right electrooculogram (LEOG, REOG) (underlined)

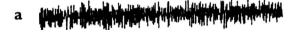

a

Figure 4.11 a, Elevated tonic digastric (submental) electromyogram (EMG). b, Low/absent tonic digastric (submental) EMG

b

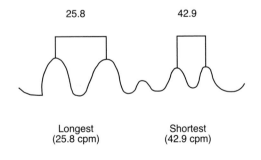

25.8   42.9

Longest   Shortest
(25.8 cpm)   (42.9 cpm)

Regular (difference < 20)

Figure 4.12 Regular/irregular respiratory rate calculation based on peak-to-peak distance measurement for the shortest and longest distances. In this example the difference is < 20, and therefore, it is considered 'regular'

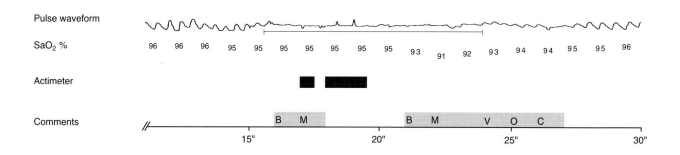

Figure 4.13 Identification of movement by the highlighted comments of BM and VOC indicating body movement and vocalization, respectively, and by the actimeter sensor marker (shown by black bars). The loss of the pulse waveform signal (underlined) is an indirect indication of movement. SaO_2 % is the oxygen saturation percent values

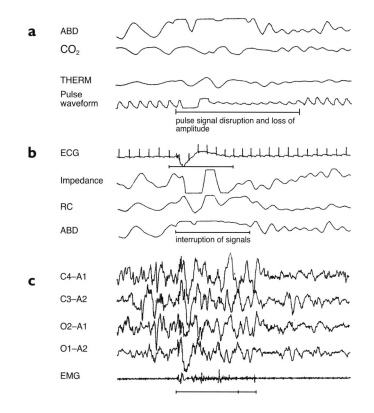

Figure 4.14 Indirect indicators of movement (underlined): a, loss of the oximeter pulse waveform artifact and blocking of abdominal (ABD) respiration; b, electrocardiogram (ECG) artifact and blocking in the impedance, rib cage (RC) and abdominal (ABD) respiratory channels; c, phasic electromyogram (EMG) burst (underlined) associated with delta waves in the electroencephalogram (C4–A1 to O1–A2)

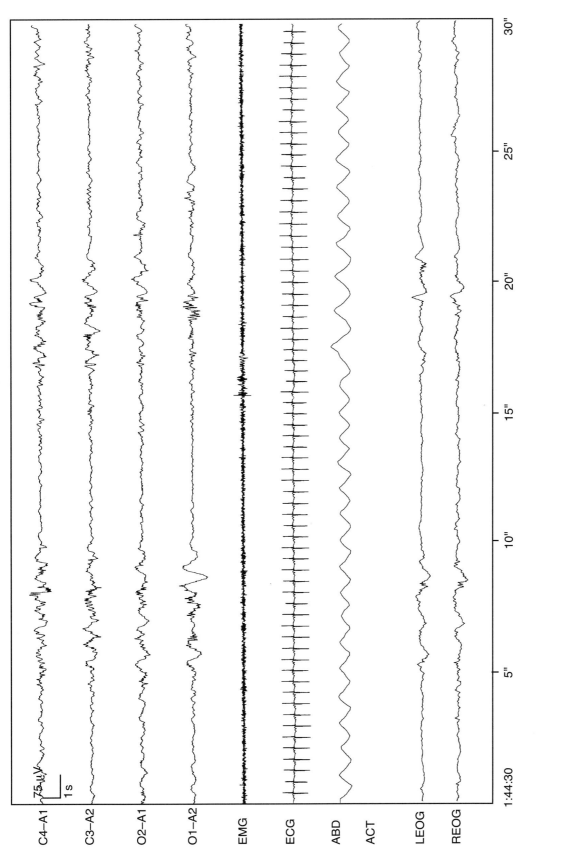

Figure 4.15 Quiet sleep in an infant of 29 weeks' gestational age, 37 weeks' conceptional age based on: no rapid eye movements in left and right electrooculogram (LEOG, REOG), tracé alternant electroencephalogram (C4–A1 to O1–A2) pattern, relatively elevated tonic submental electromyogram (EMG), regular abdominal (ABD) respiration and no body movement in the actimeter (ACT) channel or comments, that is, five of five quiet sleep parameters

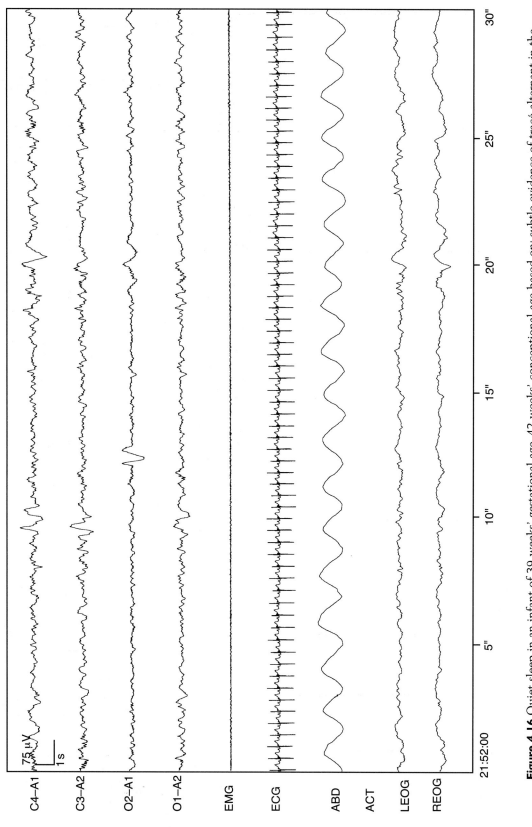

Figure 4.16 Quiet sleep in an infant of 39 weeks' gestational age, 42 weeks' conceptional age based on: subtle evidence of tracé alternant in the electroencephalogram (C4–A1, C3–A2), regular abdominal (ABD) respiration, no rapid eye movements in the left and right electrooculogram (LEOG, REOG), no body movements in the actimeter (ACT) and no comments. Submental electromyogram (EMG) appears to have a low tonic level (an active sleep condition), but this must be evaluated relative to this infant's tonic levels throughout the night. If no changes are discernible, the EMG may need to be eliminated from the state decision. This would result in four of four or four of five quiet sleep parameters. O2–A1, O1–A2, electrooculogram; ECG, electrocardiogram

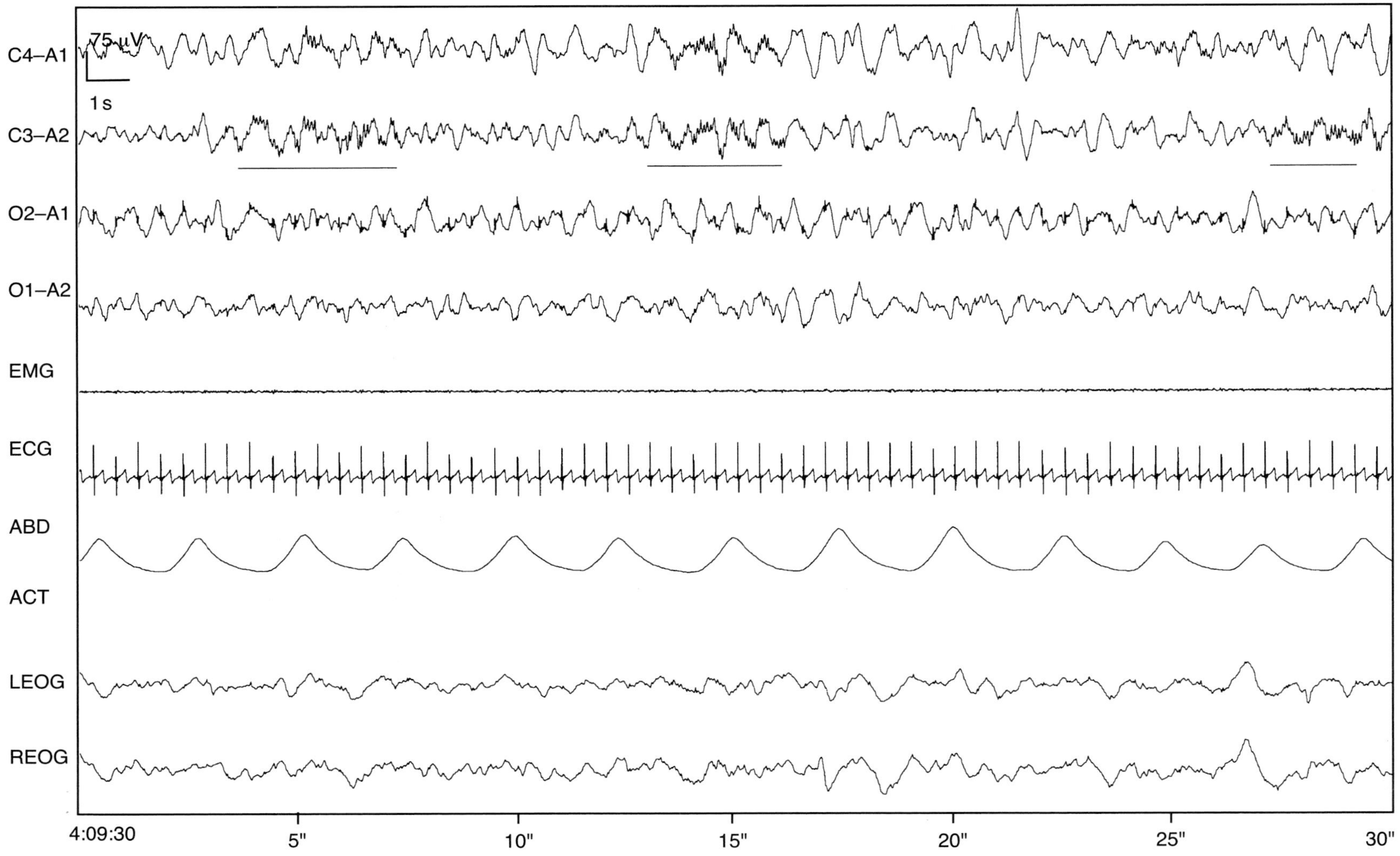

Figure 4.17 Quiet sleep in an infant of 39 weeks' gestational age, 48 weeks' conceptional age based on: relatively high-voltage slow electroencephalogram (C4–A1 to O1–A2) (> 50 µV for > 50% of the epoch) with evidence of sleep spindles (see underline in C3–A2), regular abdominal (ABD) respiration, no rapid eye movements in left and right electrooculogram (LEOG, REOG), no body movements in the actimeter (ACT) and no comments. The tonic electromyogram (EMG) does not meet quiet sleep criteria. Depending on the EMG status this result would be four of four or four of five quiet sleep parameters. ECG, electrocardiogram

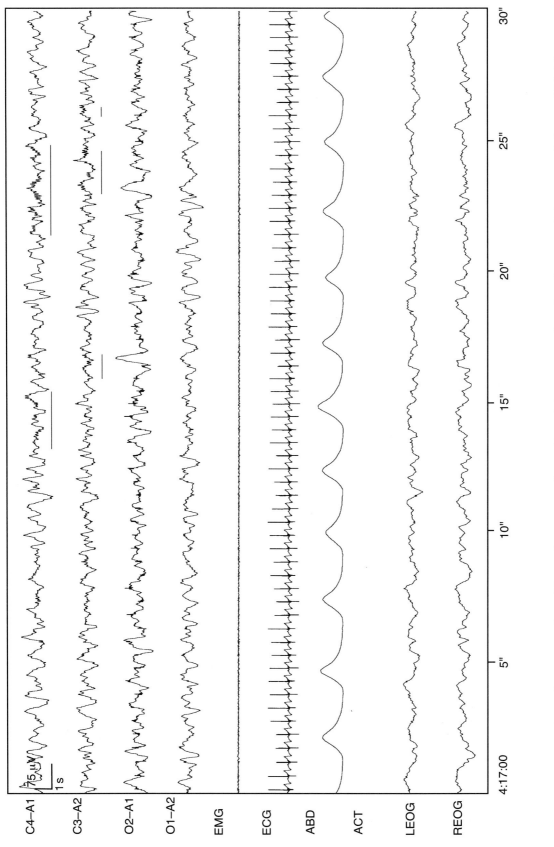

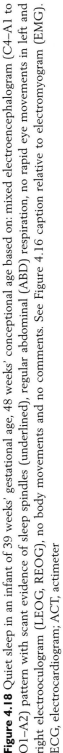

Figure 4.18 Quiet sleep in an infant of 39 weeks' gestational age, 48 weeks' conceptional age based on: mixed electroencephalogram (C4–A1 to O1–A2) pattern with scant evidence of sleep spindles (underlined), regular abdominal (ABD) respiration, no rapid eye movements in left and right electrooculogram (LEOG, REOG), no body movements and no comments. See Figure 4.16 caption relative to electromyogram (EMG). ECG, electrocardiogram; ACT, actimeter

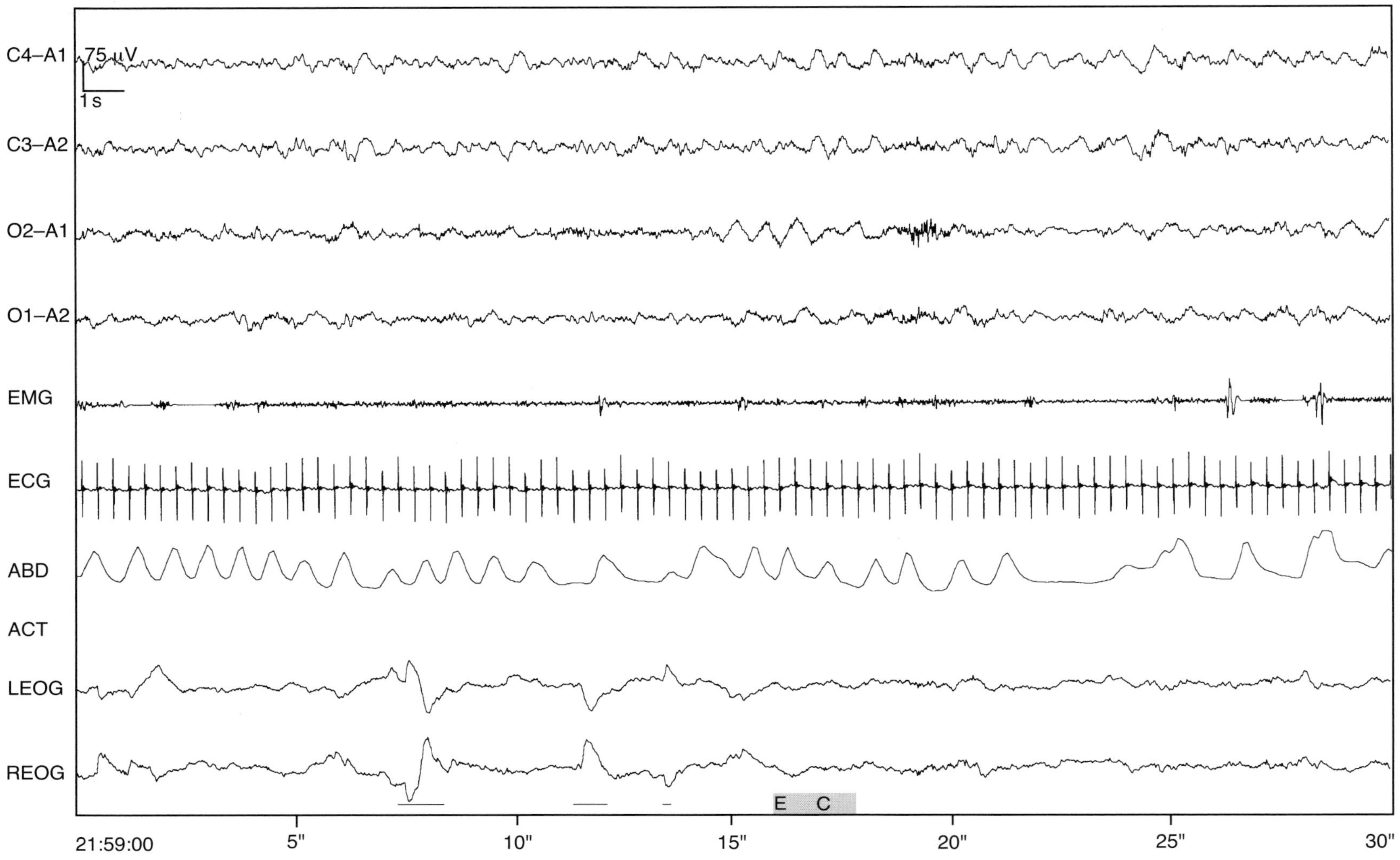

Figure 4.19 Active sleep in an infant of 29 weeks' gestational age, 34 weeks' conceptional age based on: presence of rapid eye movements (see underlines below the right electrooculogram (REOG) channel), mixed electroencephalogram (C4–A1 to O1–A2) pattern, irregular abdominal (ABD) respiration. There is no annotation of body movement and the electromyogram (EMG) was not included in the state determination. The sleep state, therefore, was based on three of four active sleep parameters. ECG, electrocardiogram; ACT, actimeter; LEOG, left electrooculogram; EC, eyes closed

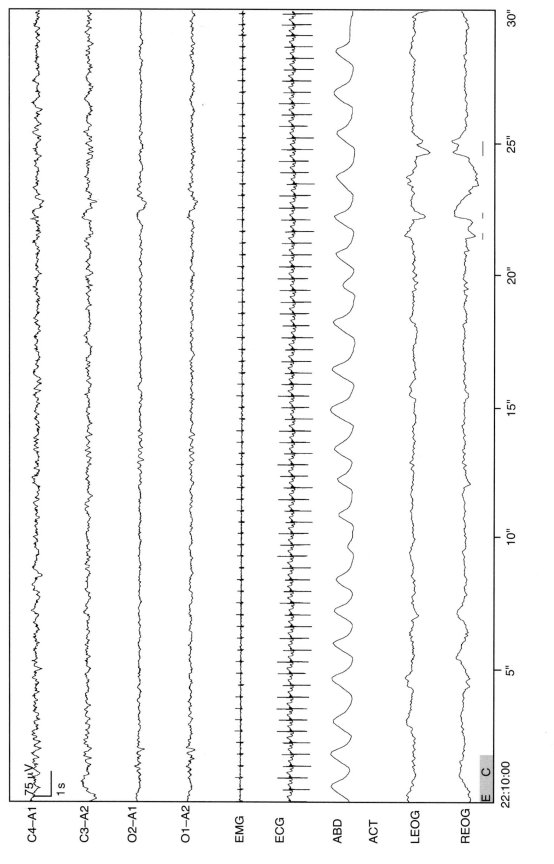

Figure 4.20 Active sleep in an infant of 39 weeks' gestational age, 42 weeks' conceptional age based on: low-voltage irregular electroencephalogram (C4–A1 to C3–A2), low tonic electromyogram (EMG) (disregarding electrocardiogram (ECG) artifact), irregular abdominal (ABD) respiration and presence of rapid eye movements in the left and right electrooculogram (LEOG, REOG) (underlined). No body movement is documented. Four of the five parameters are associated with active sleep. EC, eyes closed

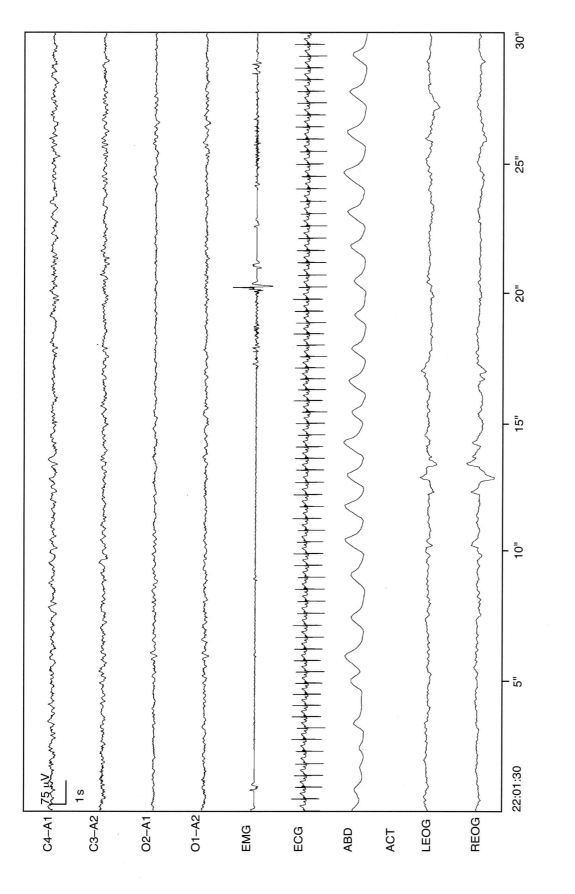

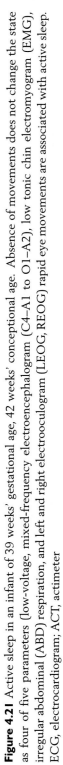

Figure 4.21 Active sleep in an infant of 39 weeks' gestational age, 42 weeks' conceptional age. Absence of movements does not change the state as four of five parameters (low-voltage, mixed-frequency electroencephalogram (C4–A1 to O1–A2), low tonic chin electromyogram (EMG), irregular abdominal (ABD) respiration, and left and right electrooculogram (LEOG, REOG) rapid eye movements are associated with active sleep. ECG, electrocardiogram; ACT, actimeter

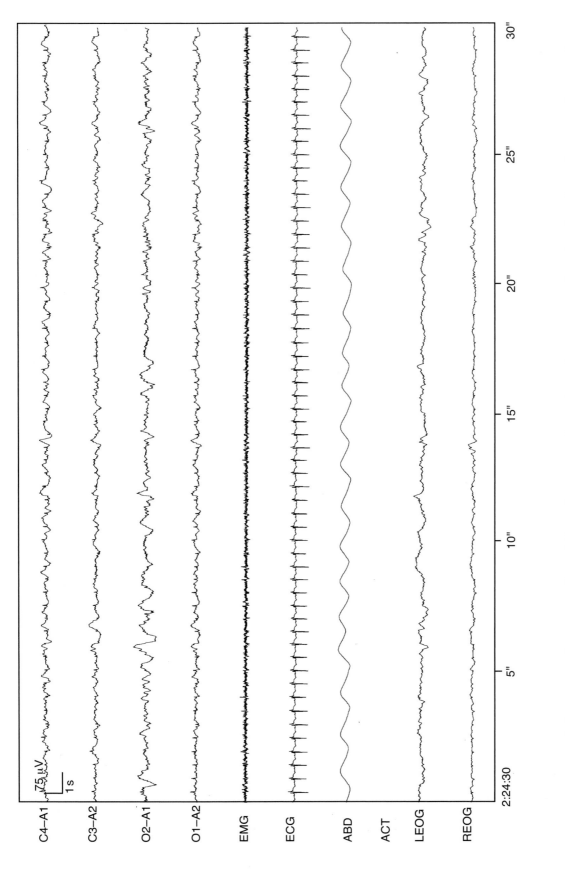

Figure 4.22 Indeterminate sleep in an infant of 40 weeks' gestational age, 41 weeks' conceptional age based on: low-voltage irregular central electroencephalogram (C4–A1, C3–A2), relatively high tonic electromyogram (EMG), regular abdominal (ABD) respiration and no rapid eye movements in the left and right electrooculogram (LEOG, REOG) or body movements in the actimeter (ACT) or comments. This is three quiet sleep and two active sleep parameters. O2–A1, O1–A2, electrooculogram; ECG, electrocardiogram

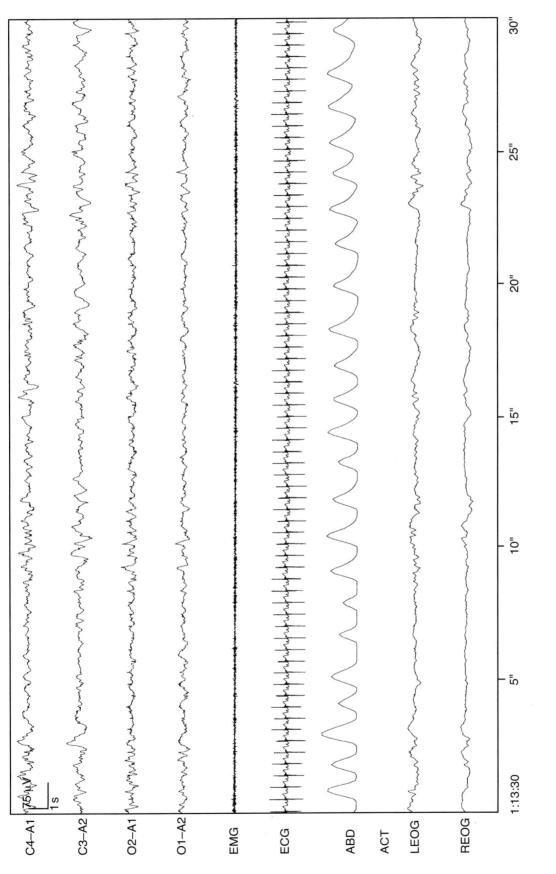

Figure 4.23 Quiet sleep in an infant of 39 weeks' gestational age, 42 weeks' conceptional age based on: transitional electroencephalogram (C4–A1 to O1–A2) pattern moving from tracé alternant to a mixed pattern between 10 and 15 s, relatively elevated tonic electromyogram (EMG), irregular abdominal (ABD) respiration, no rapid eye movements in left and right electrooculogram (LEOG, REOG), no body movements in the actimeter (ACT) channel or comments related to movements. Four of the five parameters are quiet sleep. ECG, electrocardiogram

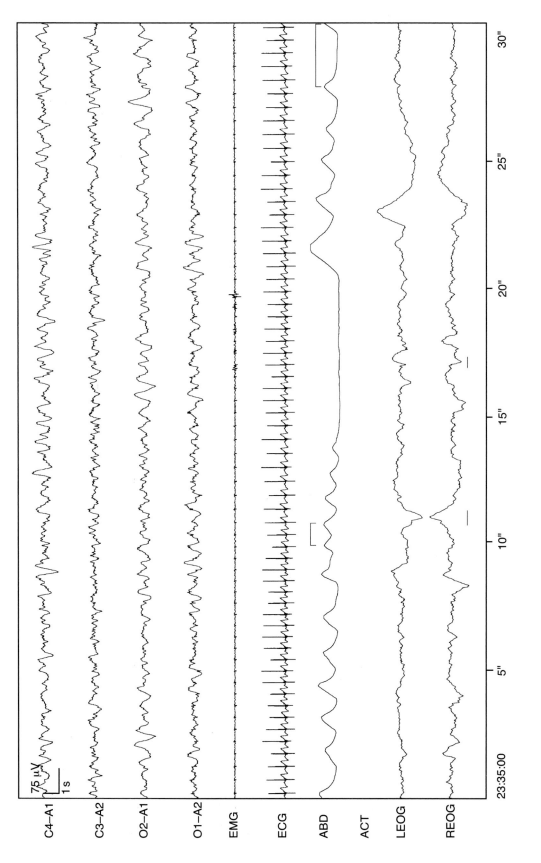

Figure 4.24 Indeterminate sleep in an infant of 39 weeks' gestational age, 48 weeks' conceptional age based on: high-voltage, slow or mixed electroencephalogram (C4–A1 to O1–A2) patterns, relatively low tonic electromyogram (EMG), irregular abdominal (ABD) respiration (shortest and longest cycles in brackets), presence of rapid eye movements in left and right electrooculogram (LEOG, REOG; underlined), no body movements in the actimeter (ACT) channel and no comments. Three of the five parameters are active sleep and two are quiet sleep. ECG, electrocardiogram

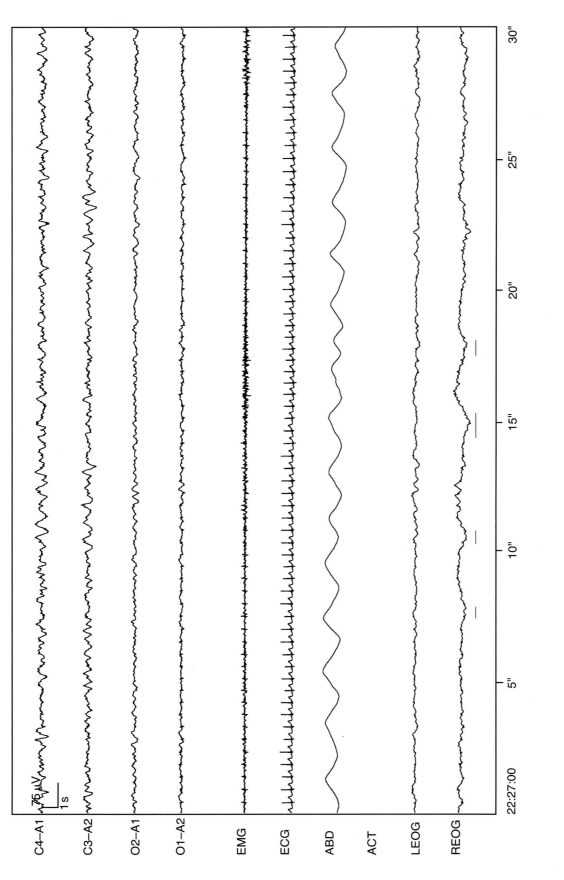

Figure 4.25 Stage 1 sleep in an infant of 40 weeks' gestational age, 51 weeks' conceptional age based on: absence of rapid eye movements in the left and right electrooculogram (LEOG, REOG) and some slight evidence of slow eye movements (underlined) with no sleep spindles in the electroencephalogram (C4–A1 to O1–A2). The tonic electromyogram (EMG) is difficult to assess in this single epoch but does show sucking bursts as increases in EMG amplitude. ABD, abdominal respiration; ACT, actimeter

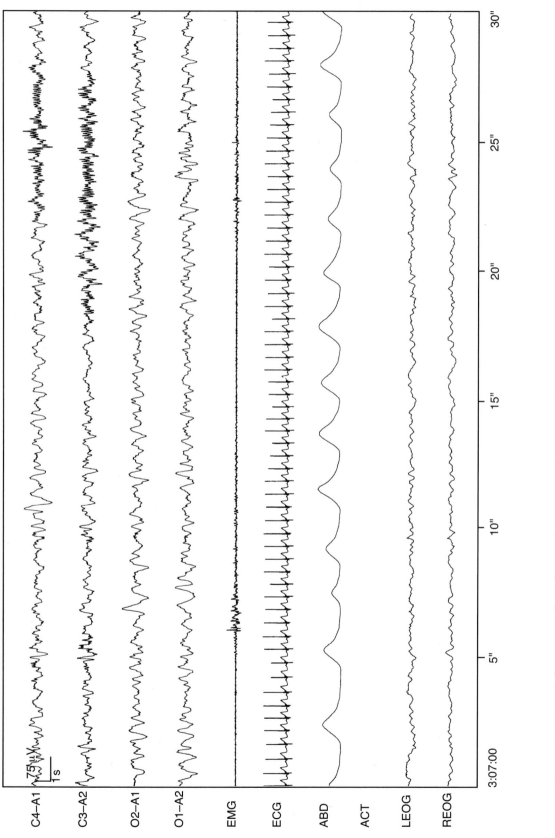

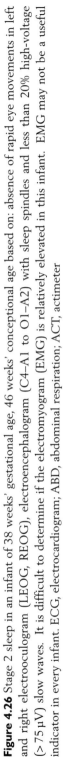

Figure 4.26 Stage 2 sleep in an infant of 38 weeks' gestational age, 46 weeks' conceptional age based on: absence of rapid eye movements in left and right electrooculogram (LEOG, REOG), electroencephalogram (C4–A1 to O1–A2) with sleep spindles and less than 20% high-voltage (>75 µV) slow waves. It is difficult to determine if the electromyogram (EMG) is relatively elevated in this infant. EMG may not be a useful indicator in every infant. ECG, electrocardiogram; ABD, abdominal respiration; ACT, actimeter

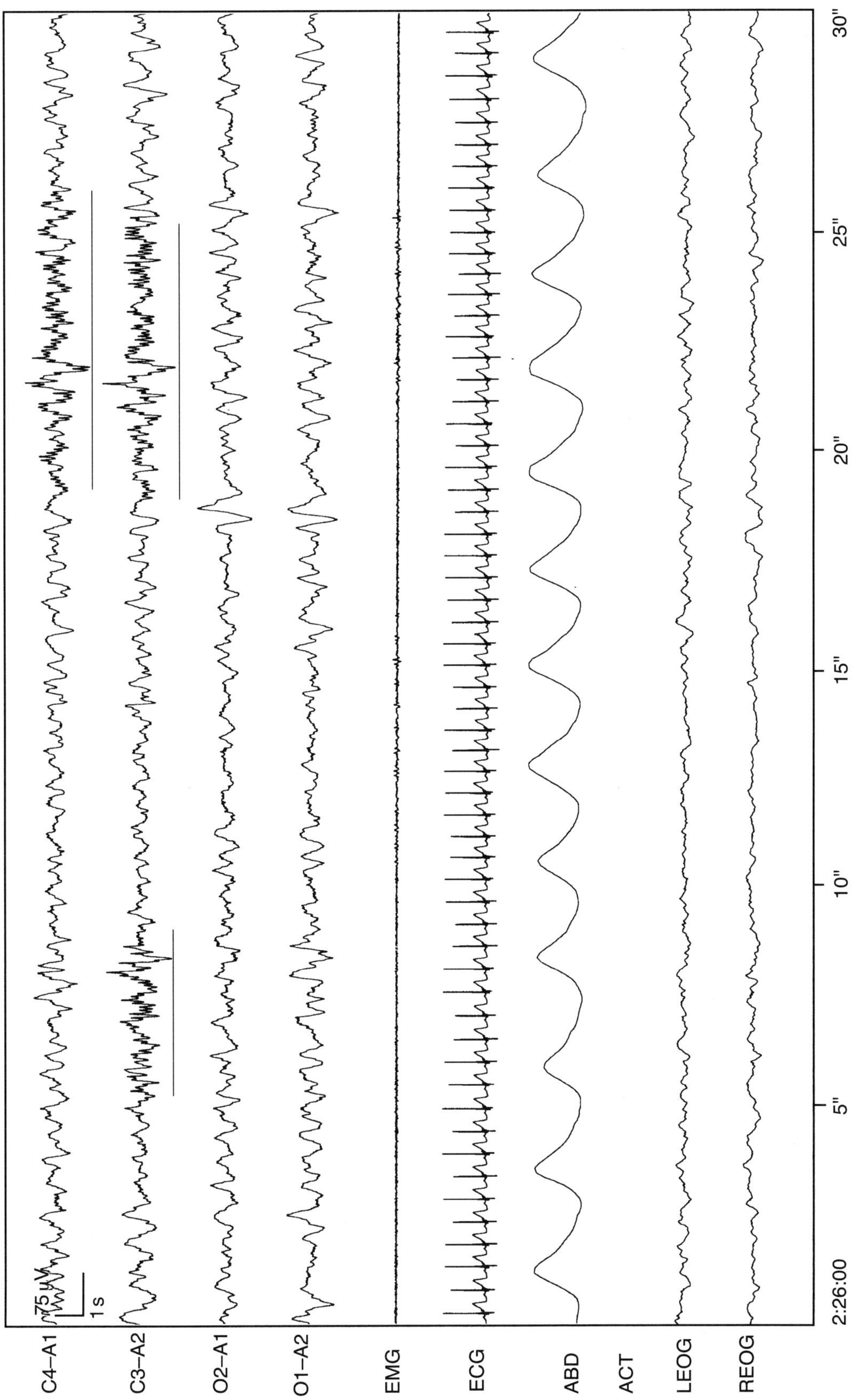

Figure 4.27 Stage 2 sleep in an infant of 38 weeks' gestational age, 46 weeks' conceptional age based on absence of rapid eye movements in the left and right electrooculogram (LEOG, REOG), presence of sleep spindles (underlined) in the electroencephalogram (C4–A1, C3–A2), and questionably elevated tonic electromyogram (EMG). The long duration of the sleep spindles with some asymmetry, that is, spindles in C3–A2 but not in C4–A1, is characteristic of this age group. ECG, electrocardiogram; ABD, abdominal respiration; ACT, actimeter

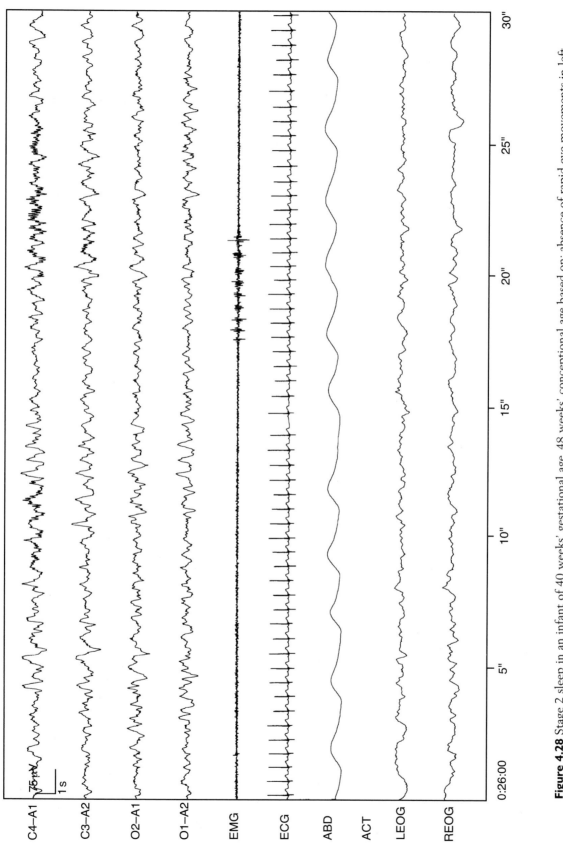

Figure 4.28 Stage 2 sleep in an infant of 40 weeks' gestational age, 48 weeks' conceptional age based on: absence of rapid eye movements in left and right electrooculogram (LEOG, REOG), presence of sleep spindles in the electroencephalogram (C4–A1), less than 20% high-voltage slow (>75 μV) waves and relatively elevated tonic electromyogram (EMG). C3–A2, O2–A1, O1–A2, electroencephalogram; ECG, electrocardiogram; ABD, abdominal respiration

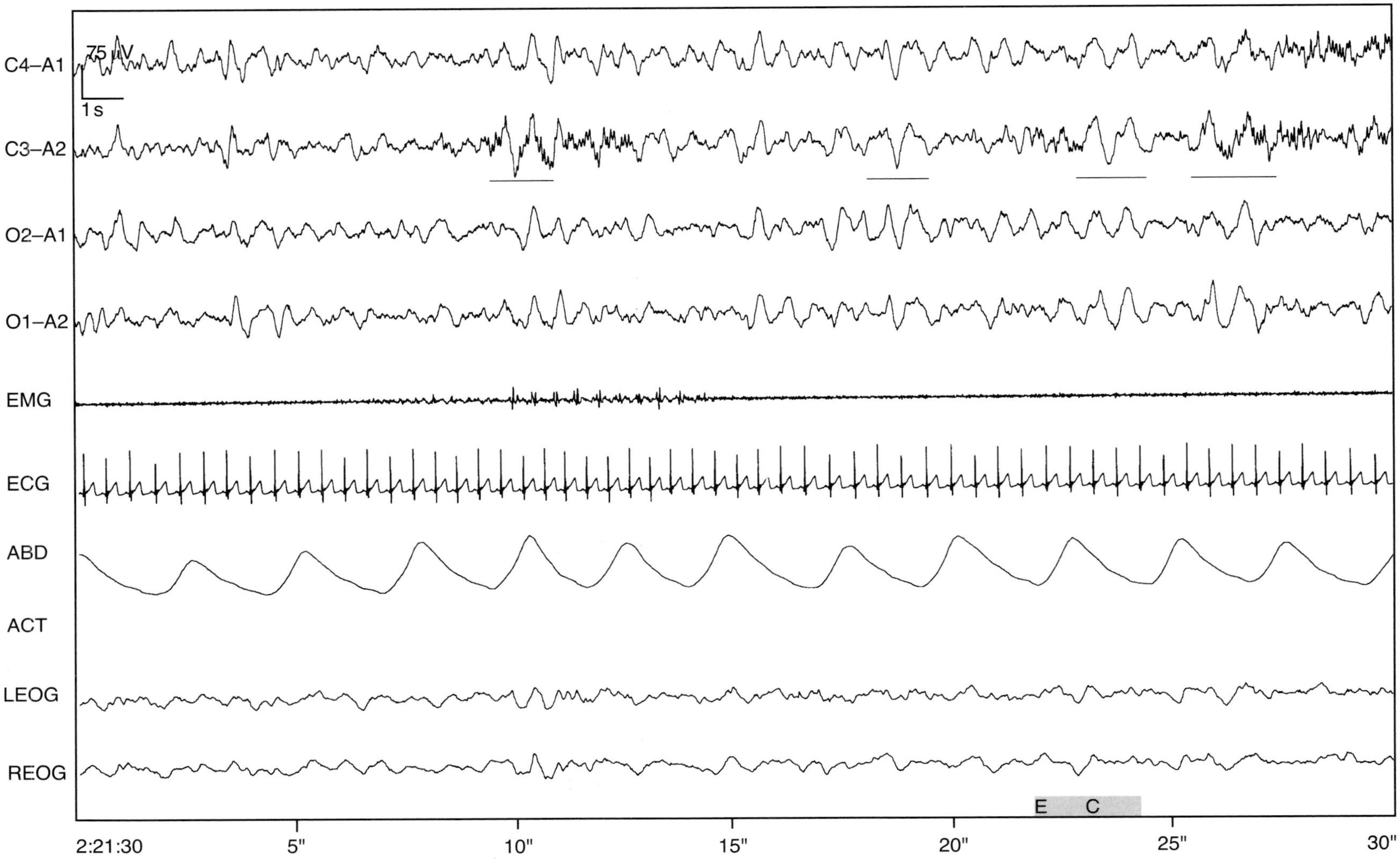

Figure 4.29 Stage 3 sleep in an infant of 38 weeks' gestational age, 46 weeks' conceptional age based on: absence of rapid eye movements in the left and right electrooculogram (LEOG, REOG), presence of sleep spindles in the electroencephalogram (C4–A1, C3–A2) and 20–50% of high-voltage (>75 μV) EEG (underlined) with relatively elevated electromyogram (EMG). O2–A1, O1–A2, electroencephalogram; ECG, electrocardiogram; ABD, abdominal respiration; ACT, actimeter; EC, eyes closed

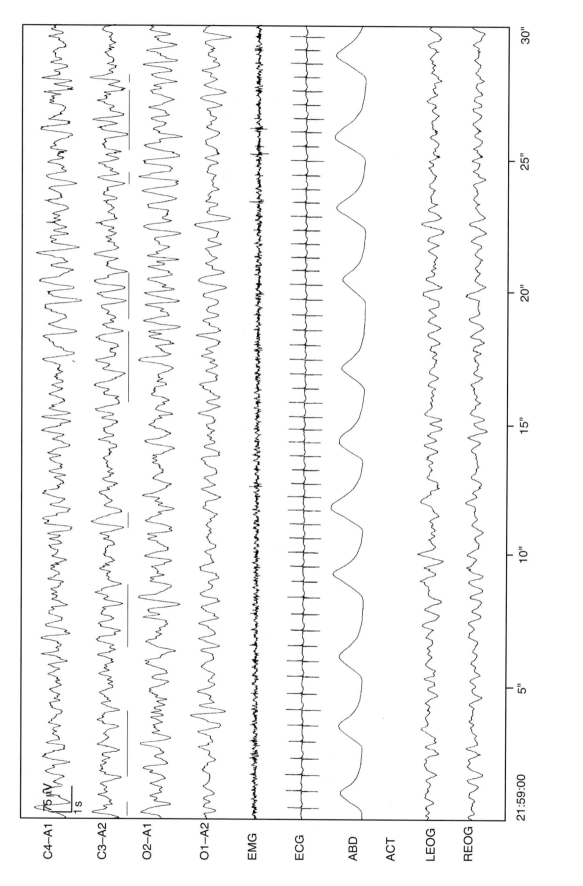

Figure 4.30 Stage 3 sleep in an infant of 39 weeks' gestational age, 52 weeks' conceptional age based on: absence of rapid eye movements in the left and right electrooculogram (LEOG, REOG), high-voltage (>75 μV) slow waves in >20% but <50% of the electroencephalogram (C4–A1 to O1–A2) (underlined), relatively elevated EMG. ECG, electrocardiogram; ABD, abdominal respiration; ACT, actimeter

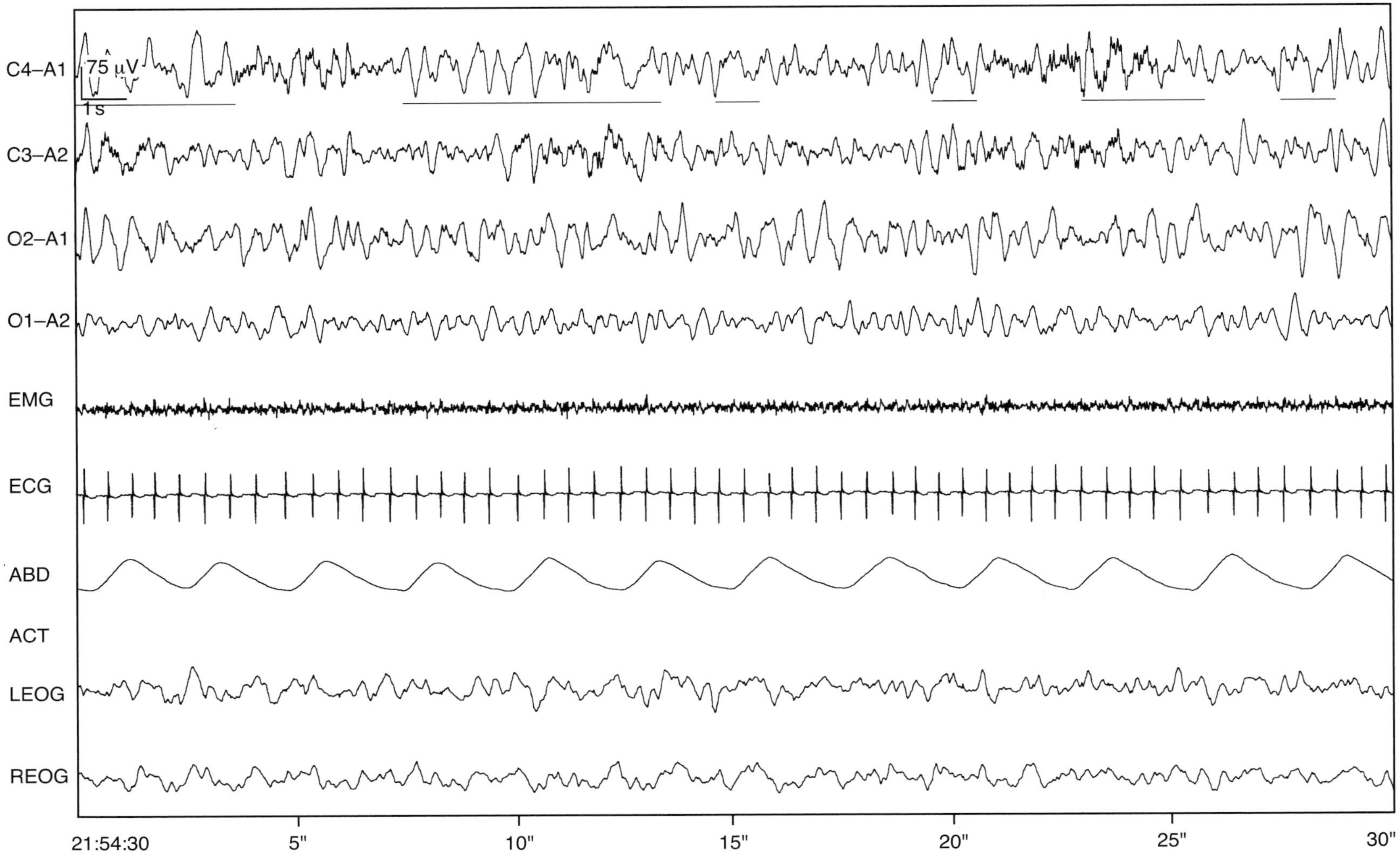

Figure 4.31 Stage 4 sleep in an infant of 39 weeks' gestational age, 48 weeks' conceptional age based on: high-voltage slow waves (>75 μV) in >50% of the electroencephalogram (C4–A1; underlined) and absence of rapid eye movements in the left and right electrooculogram (LEOG, REOG). The tonic electromyogram (EMG) level appears to be relatively elevated. C3–A2, O1–A2, electroencephalogram; ECG, electrocardiogram; ABD, abdominal respiration; O2–A1, O1–A2, electroencephalogram; ACT, actimeter

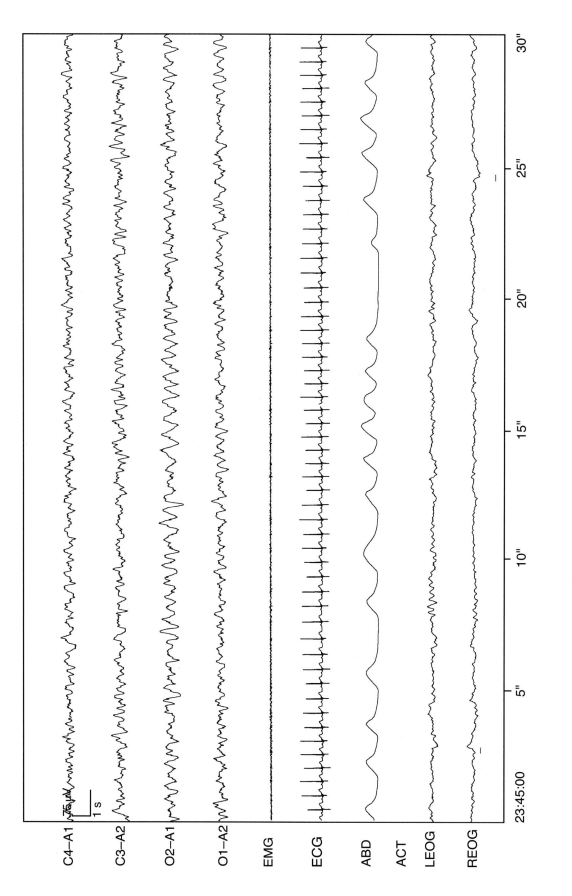

Figure 4.32 Stage REM sleep in an infant of 40 weeks' gestational age, 48 weeks' conceptional age based on presence of rapid eye movements in the left and right electrooculogram (LEOG, REOG; underlined), low-voltage irregular electroencephalogram (C4–A1, C3–A2) and relatively low tonic submental electromyogram (EMG). Although not part of the adult scoring criteria, irregular abdominal (ABD) respiration and irregular heart rate in the electrocardiogram (ECG) channel are also present. O2–A1, O1–A2, electroencephalogram; ACT, actimeter

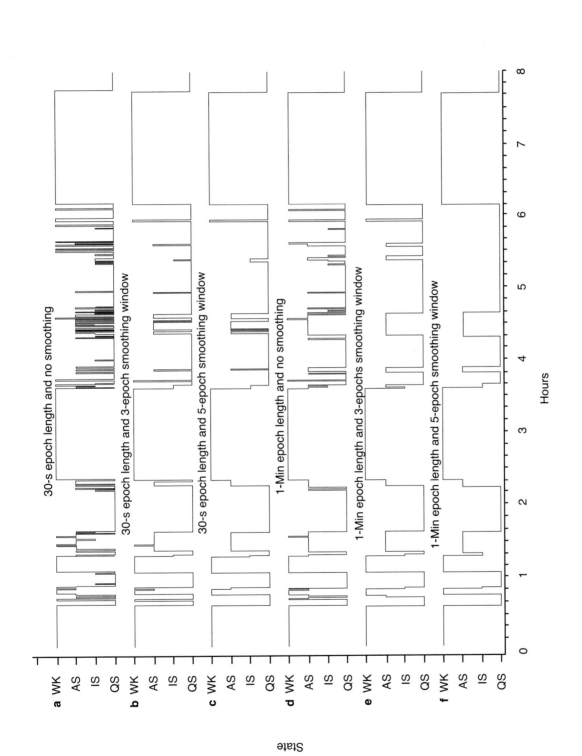

Figure 4.33 Infant polysomnography sleep architecture of a single infant illustrating the smoothing process applied to both epoch length (30 s or 1 min) and smoothing window (none, 3 epochs, 5 epochs) as shown in Panels a–f. WK, wake; AS, active sleep; IS, indeterminate sleep; QS, quiet sleep

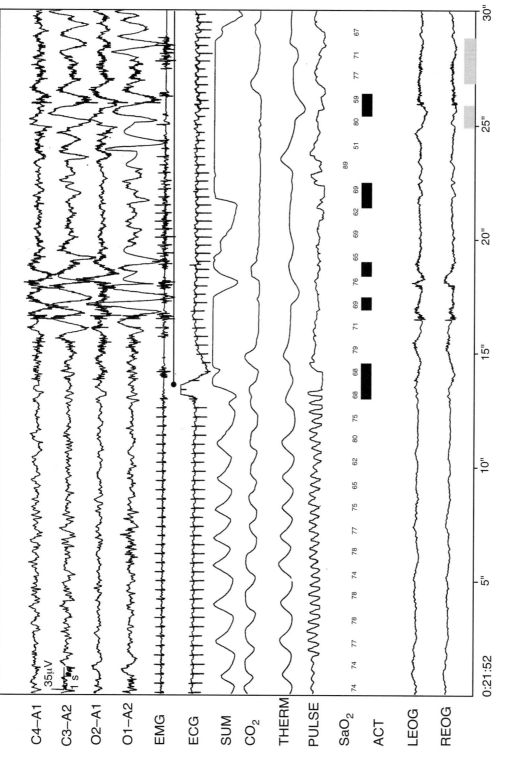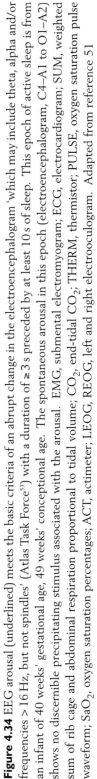

Figure 4.34 EEG arousal (underlined) meets the basic criteria of an abrupt change in the electroencephalogram 'which may include theta, alpha and/or frequencies > 16 Hz, but not spindles' (Atlas Task Force[53]) with a duration of ≥3 s preceded by at least 10 s of sleep. This epoch of active sleep is from an infant of 40 weeks' gestational age, 49 weeks' conceptional age. The spontaneous arousal in this epoch shows no discernible precipitating stimulus associated with the arousal. EMG, submental electromyogram; ECG, electrocardiogram; SUM, weighted sum of rib cage and abdominal respiration proportional to tidal volume; CO_2, end-tidal CO_2; THERM, thermistor; PULSE, oxygen saturation pulse waveform; SaO_2, oxygen saturation percentages; ACT, actimeter; LEOG, REOG, left and right electrooculogram. Adapted from reference 51

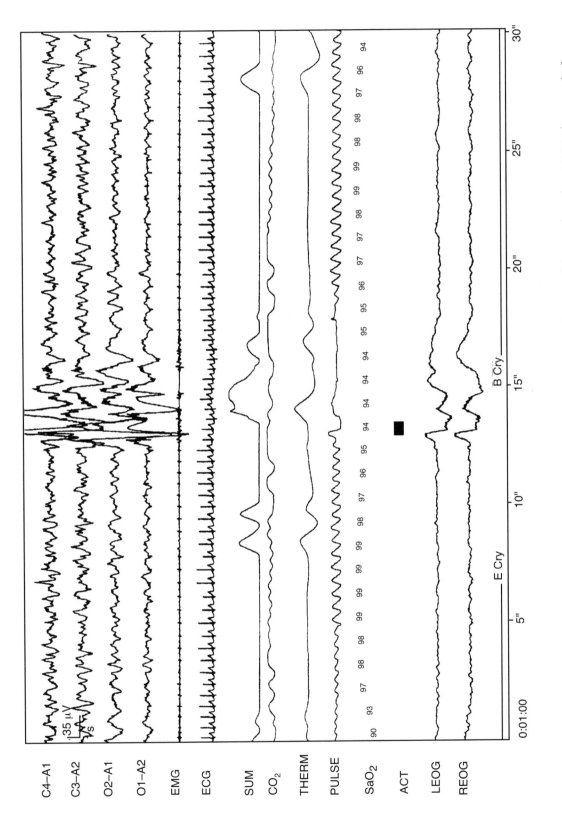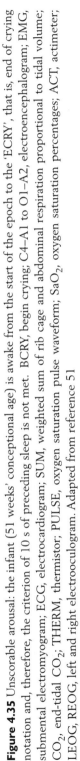

Figure 4.35 Unscorable arousal: the infant (51 weeks' conceptional age) is awake from the start of the epoch to the 'ECRY', that is, end of crying notation and, therefore, the criterion of 10 s of preceding sleep is not met. BCRY, begin crying; C4–A1 to O1–A2, electroencephalogram; EMG, submental electromyogram; ECG, electrocardiogram; SUM, weighted sum of rib cage and abdominal respiration proportional to tidal volume; CO_2, end-tidal CO_2; THERM, thermistor; PULSE, oxygen saturation pulse waveform; SaO_2, oxygen saturation percentages; ACT, actimeter; LEOG, REOG, left and right electrooculogram. Adapted from reference 51

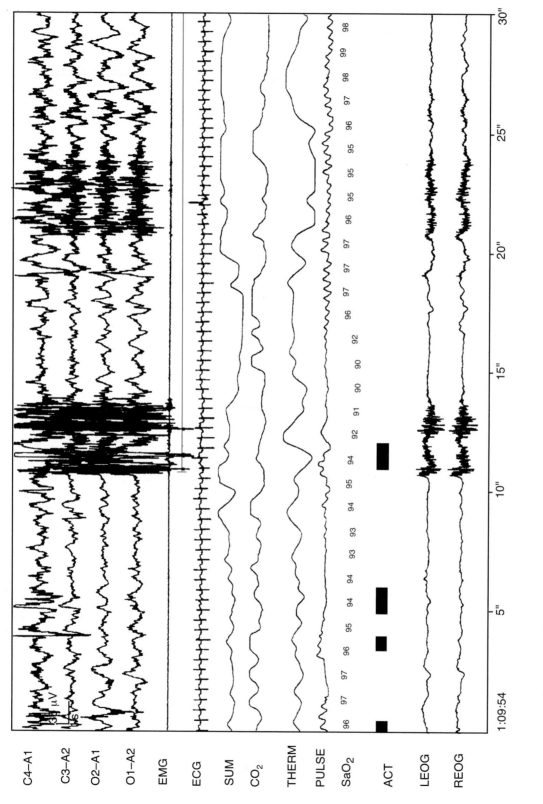

Figure 4.36 Infant (35 weeks' conceptional age): two arousals occur without 10 s of sleep preceding the second; therefore, the two are scored as one arousal (underlined). C4–A1 to O1–A2, electroencephalogram; EMG, submental electromyogram; ECG, electrocardiogram; SUM, weighted sum of rib cage and abdominal respiration proportional to tidal volume; CO_2, end tidal CO_2; THERM, thermistor; PULSE, oxygen saturation pulse waveform; ACT, actimeter; LEOG, REOG, left and right electrooculogram; SaO_2, oxygen saturation percentages. Adapted from reference 51

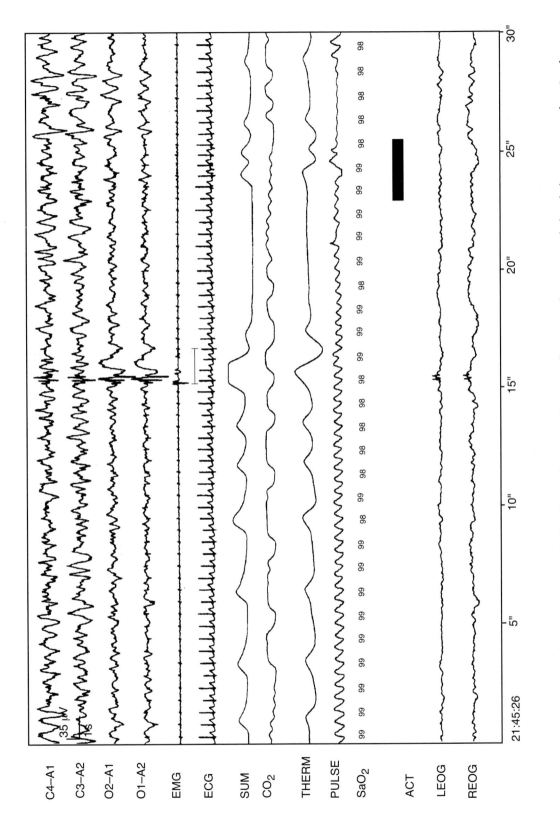

Figure 4.37 Infant (51 weeks' conceptional age): the abrupt electroencephalogram frequency change, as underlined, does not meet the ≥3-s duration criterion, and therefore, cannot be scored as an arousal. C4–A1 to O1–A2, electroencephalogram; EMG, submental electromyogram; ECG, electrocardiogram; SUM, weighted sum of rib cage and abdominal respiration proportional to tidal volume; CO_2, end-tidal CO_2; THERM, thermistor; PULSE, oxygen saturation pulse waveform; SaO_2, oxygen saturation percentages; ACT, actimeter; LEOG, REOG, left and right electrooculogram. Adapted from reference 51

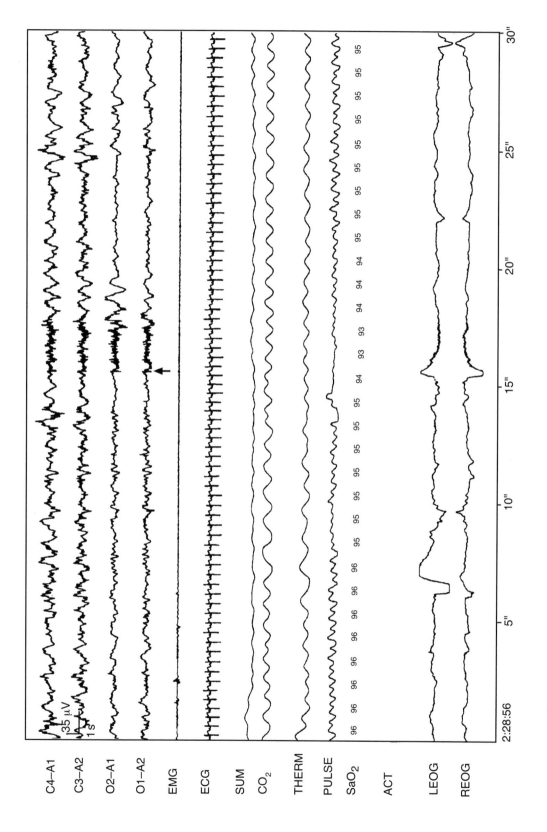

Figure 4.38 Infant (51 weeks' conceptional age): in active sleep, the electroencephalogram frequency shift that meets arousal criteria (arrow) must be accompanied by a concurrent increase in electromyogram (EMG) amplitude, which is not seen in this epoch. Delta activity occurring prior to the frequency shift would not be included in any arousal duration. No arousal was scored for this epoch. C4–A1 to O1–A2, electroencephalogram; EMG, submental EMG; ECG, electrocardiogram; SUM, weighted sum of rib cage and abdominal respiration proportional to tidal volume; CO_2, end-tidal CO_2; THERM, thermistor; PULSE, oxygen saturation pulse waveform; SaO_2, oxygen saturation percentages; ACT, actimeter; LEOG, REOG, left and right electrooculogram. Adapted from reference 51

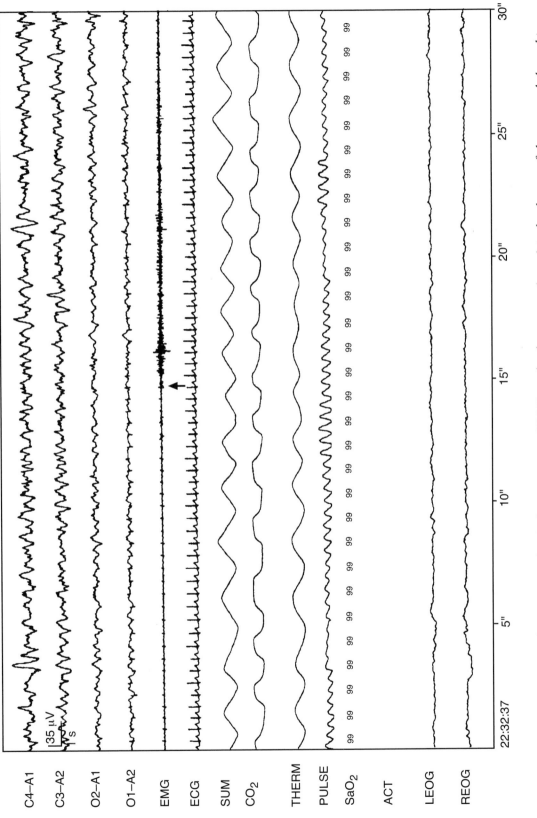
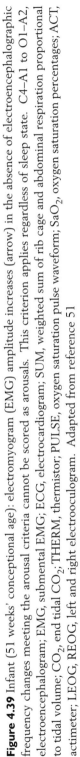

Figure 4.39 Infant (51 weeks' conceptional age): electromyogram (EMG) amplitude increases (arrow) in the absence of electroencephalographic frequency changes meeting the arousal criteria cannot be scored as arousals. This criterion applies regardless of sleep state. C4–A1 to O1–A2, electroencephalogram; EMG, submental EMG; ECG, electrocardiogram; SUM, weighted sum of rib cage and abdominal respiration proportional to tidal volume; CO_2, end tidal CO_2; THERM, thermistor; PULSE, oxygen saturation pulse waveform; SaO_2, oxygen saturation percentages; ACT, actimeter; LEOG, REOG, left and right electrooculogram. Adapted from reference 51

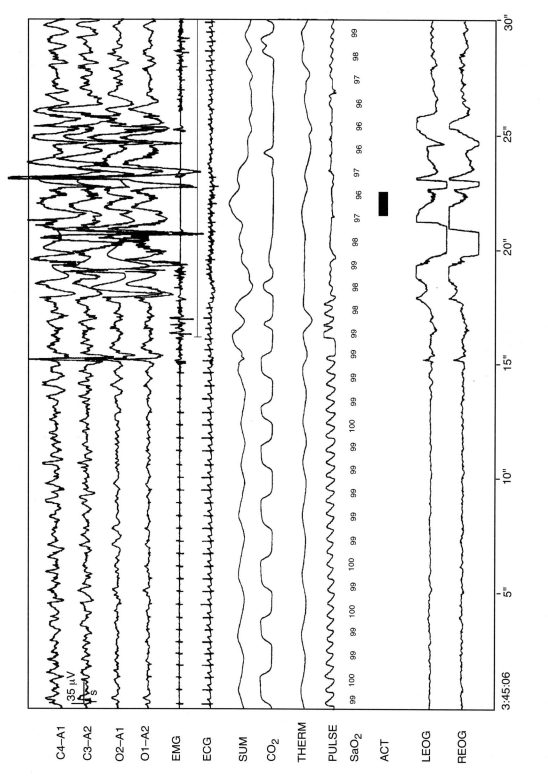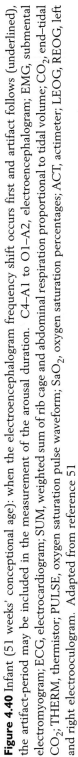

Figure 4.40 Infant (51 weeks' conceptional age): when the electroencephalogram frequency shift occurs first and artifact follows (underlined), the artifact-period may be included in the measurement of the arousal duration. C4–A1 to O1–A2, electroencephalogram; EMG, submental electromyogram; ECG, electrocardiogram; SUM, weighted sum of rib cage and abdominal respiration proportional to tidal volume; CO₂, end-tidal CO₂; THERM, thermistor; PULSE, oxygen saturation pulse waveform; SaO₂, oxygen saturation percentages; ACT, actimeter; LEOG, REOG, left and right electrooculogram. Adapted from reference 51

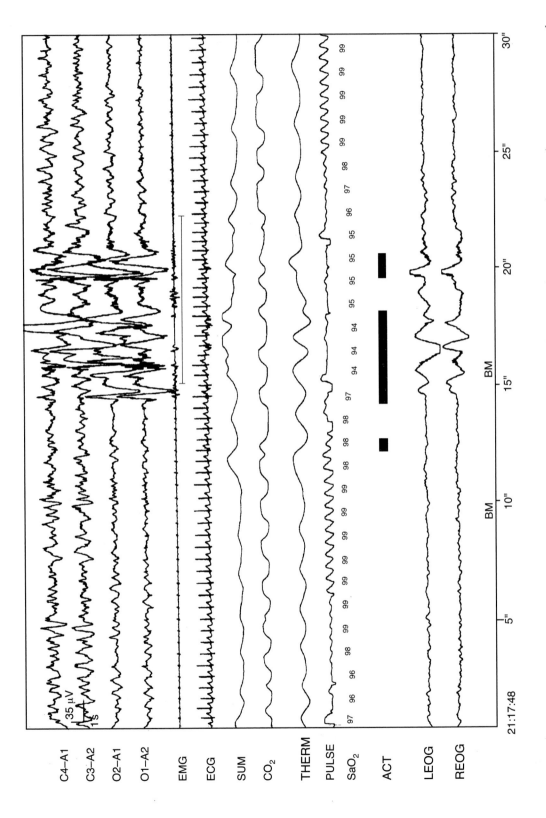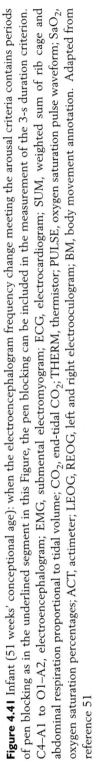

Figure 4.41 Infant (51 weeks' conceptional age): when the electroencephalogram frequency change meeting the arousal criteria contains periods of pen blocking as in the underlined segment in this Figure, the pen blocking can be included in the measurement of the 3-s duration criterion. C4–A1 to O1–A2, electroencephalogram; EMG, submental electromyogram; ECG, electrocardiogram; SUM, weighted sum of rib cage and abdominal respiration proportional to tidal volume; CO_2, end-tidal CO_2; THERM, thermistor; PULSE, oxygen saturation pulse waveform; SaO_2, oxygen saturation percentages; ACT, actimeter; LEOG, REOG, left and right electrooculogram; BM, body movement annotation. Adapted from reference 51

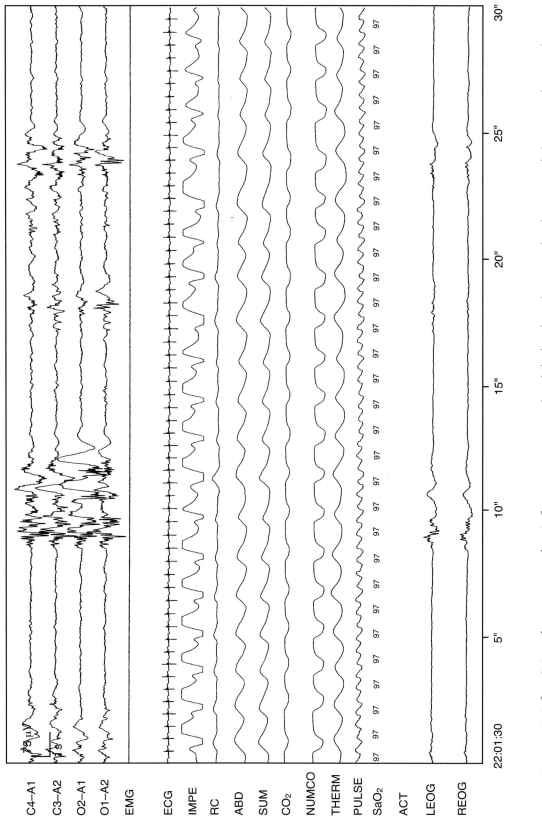

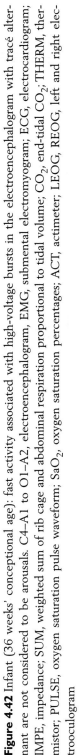

Figure 4.42 Infant (36 weeks' conceptional age): fast activity associated with high-voltage bursts in the electroencephalogram with tracé alternant are not considered to be arousals. C4–A1 to O1–A2, electroencephalogram, EMG, submental electromyogram; ECG, electrocardiogram; IMPE, impedance; SUM, weighted sum of rib cage and abdominal respiration proportional to tidal volume; CO_2, end-tidal CO_2; THERM, thermistor; PULSE, oxygen saturation pulse waveform; SaO_2, oxygen saturation percentages; ACT, actimeter; LEOG, REOG, left and right electrooculogram

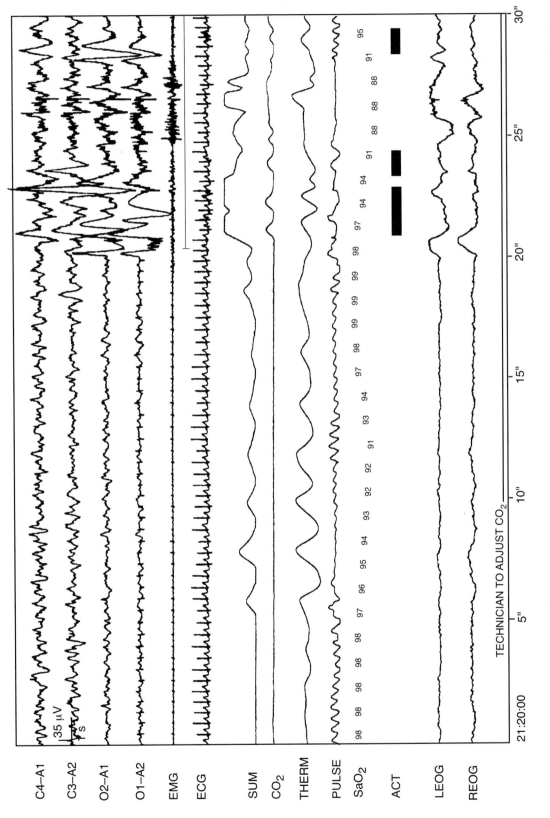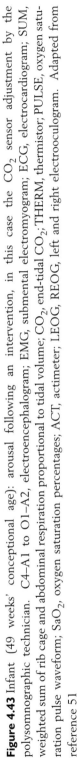

Figure 4.43 Infant (49 weeks' conceptional age): arousal following an intervention, in this case the CO_2 sensor adjustment by the polysomnographic technician. C4–A1 to O1–A2, electroencephalogram; EMG, submental electromyogram; ECG, electrocardiogram; SUM, weighted sum of rib cage and abdominal respiration proportional to tidal volume; CO_2, end-tidal CO_2; THERM, thermistor; PULSE, oxygen saturation pulse waveform; SaO_2, oxygen saturation percentages; ACT, actimeter; LEOG, REOG, left and right electrooculogram. Adapted from reference 51

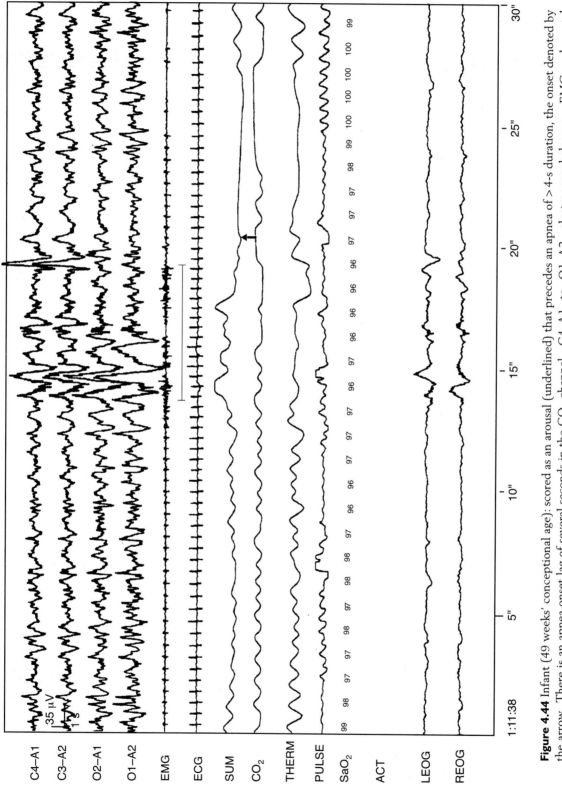

Figure 4.44 Infant (49 weeks' conceptional age): scored as an arousal (underlined) that precedes an apnea of >4-s duration, the onset denoted by the arrow. There is an apnea onset lag of several seconds in the CO_2 channel. C4–A1 to O1–A2, electroencephalogram; EMG, submental electromyogram; ECG, electrocardiogram; SUM, weighted sum of rib cage and abdominal respiration proportional to tidal volume; CO_2, end-tidal CO_2; THERM, thermistor; PULSE, oxygen saturation pulse waveform; SaO_2, oxygen saturation percentages; ACT, actimeter; LEOG, REOG, left and right electrooculogram. Adapted from reference 51

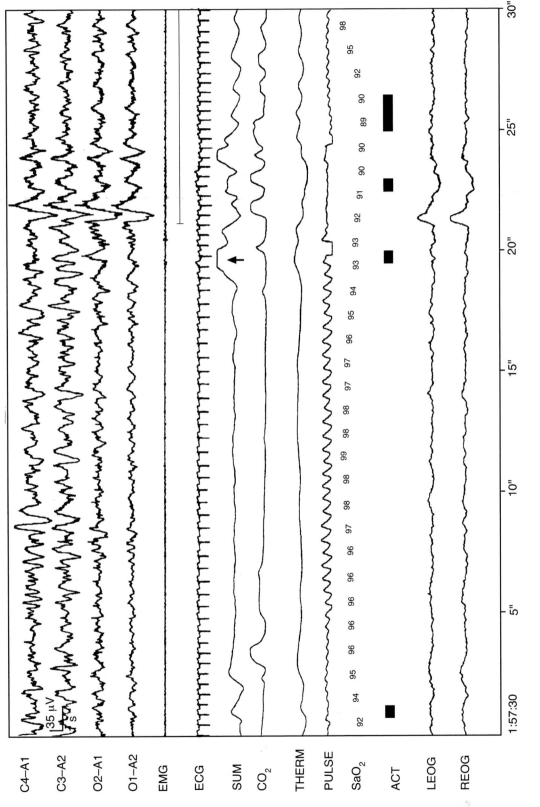

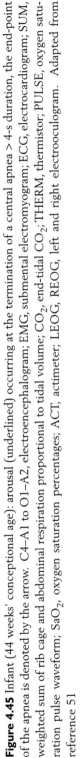

Figure 4.45 Infant (44 weeks' conceptional age): arousal (underlined) occurring at the termination of a central apnea > 4-s duration, the end-point of the apnea is denoted by the arrow. C4–A1 to O1–A2, electroencephalogram; EMG, submental electromyogram; ECG, electrocardiogram; SUM, weighted sum of rib cage and abdominal respiration proportional to tidal volume; CO_2, end-tidal CO_2; THERM, thermistor; PULSE, oxygen saturation pulse waveform; SaO_2, oxygen saturation percentages; ACT, actimeter; LEOG, REOG, left and right electrooculogram. Adapted from reference 51

a   Normal sinus rhythm

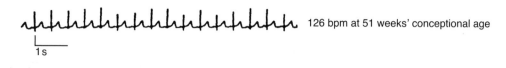

126 bpm at 51 weeks' conceptional age

1 s

b   Sinus arrhythmia

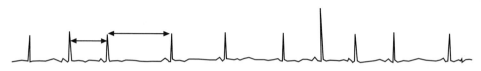

Figure 4.46 Examples of normal electrocardiogram. a, Sinus rhythm; b, sinus arrhythmia where the arrows highlight the R–R interval differences

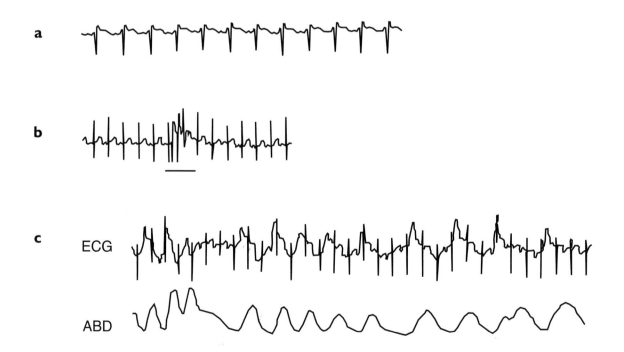

a

b

c   ECG

ABD

Figure 4.47 Examples of electrocardiogram recordings with artifacts or other problems. a, Extremely low-amplitude R-wave. b, Movement artifact (underlined). c, Baseline changes associated with breaths. ECG, electrocardiogram; ABD, abdominal respiration

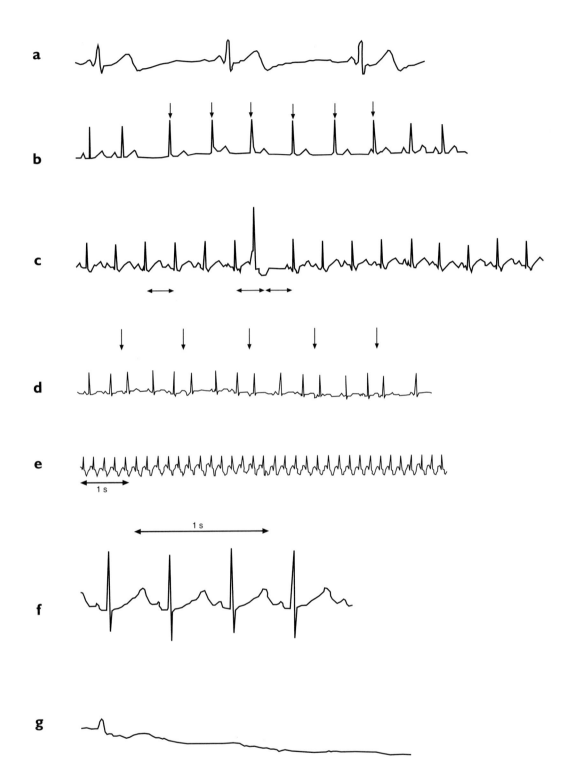

Figure 4.48 Cardiac arrhythmia examples. a, Sinus bradycardia, 45 beats/min. b, Junctional escape beats (arrows) as a function of sinus arrhythmia. Even though there is a P-wave preceding the last junctional beat, the P occurs too late to cause ventricular depolarization. c, Premature ventricular beat (PVC) is a beat that occurs earlier than expected and has a wide QRS complex. The normal sinus rhythm returns after the PVC; the time from the beat before to the beat after the PVC is twice the normal R–R interval (shown by the arrow). This timing is a hallmark of a PVC. d, Premature atrial contraction as shown by arrows. The QRS complexes are similar in form to normal beats, but they occur earlier than expected. e, Paroxysmal atrial tachycardia showing rapid rate and abnormal appearing complexes. f, Long QT intervals with a heart rate of 150 beats/min and a QT interval of 322 ms. Corrected for heart rate QT is 477 ms, which is abnormally prolonged. g, Asystole

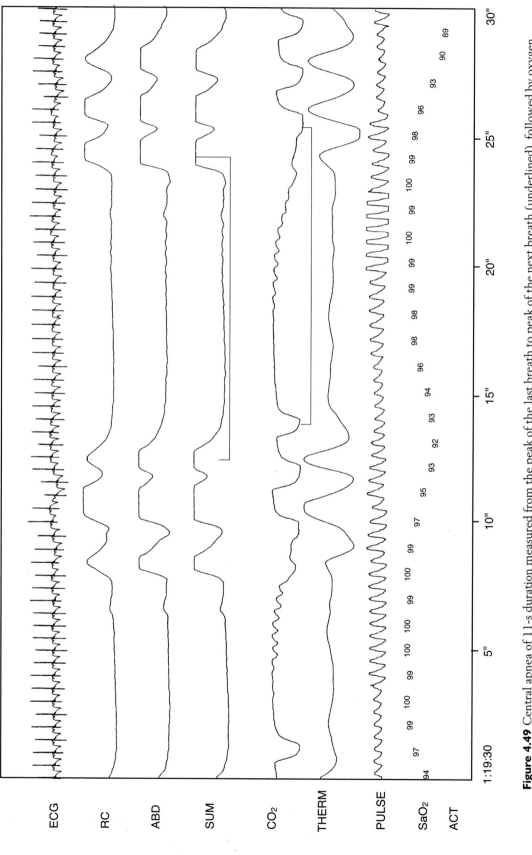
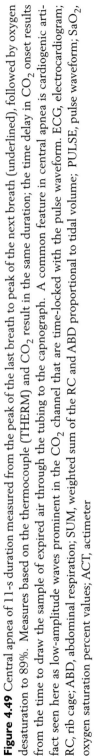

Figure 4.49 Central apnea of 11-s duration measured from the peak of the last breath to peak of the next breath (underlined), followed by oxygen desaturation to 89%. Measures based on the thermocouple (THERM) and CO_2 result in the same duration; the time delay in CO_2 onset results from the time to draw the sample of expired air through the tubing to the capnograph. A common feature in central apnea is cardiogenic artifact seen here as low-amplitude waves prominent in the CO_2 channel that are time-locked with the pulse waveform. ECG, electrocardiogram; RC, rib cage; ABD, abdominal respiration; SUM, weighted sum of the RC and ABD proportional to tidal volume; PULSE, pulse waveform; SaO_2, oxygen saturation percent values; ACT, actimeter

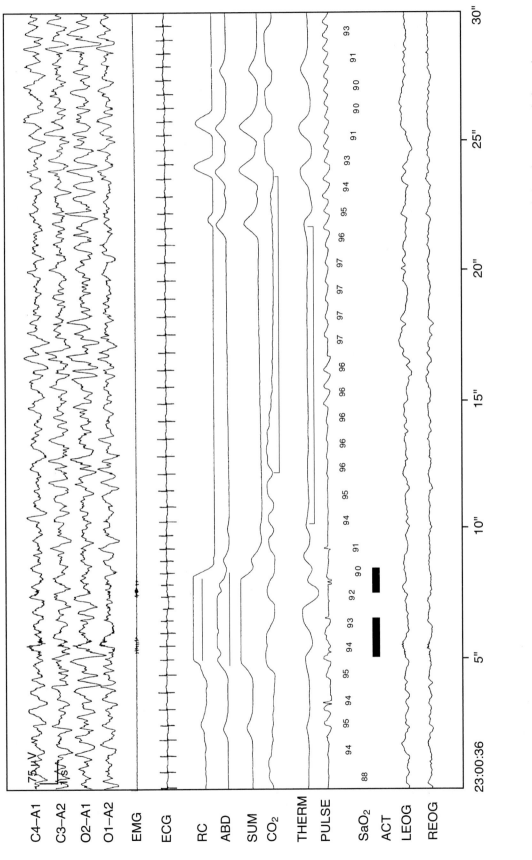

Figure 4.50 Central apnea (underlined) following movement and arousal as demonstrated by the flattening of the electroencephalographic channels (C4–A1 to O1–A2) and blocking (underlined) in the rib cage (RC) and abdominal respiration (ABD) channels; the disruption in the pulse waveform (PULSE) coincides with a movement shown by the black actimeter (ACT) bars. EMG, submental electromyogram; ECG, electrocardiogram; SUM, weighted sum of the RC and ABD proportional to tidal volume; CO_2, end-tidal CO_2; THERM, thermistor; SaO_2, oxygen saturation percent values; LEOG, REOG, left and right electrooculogram

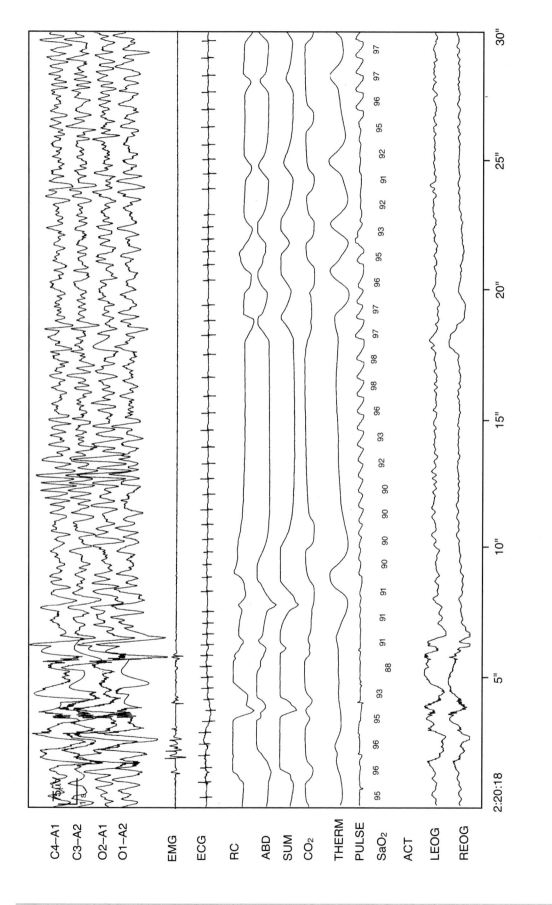

Figure 4.51 Brief central apnea following an arousal prior to 10 s. The lowest desaturation percentages that follow this event must be disregarded because the loss of the pulse waveform renders the percentages uninterpretable. Note the out-of-phase breaths in the rib cage (RC) and abdominal (ABD) respiration channels following the apneic event. C4–A1 to O1–A2, electroencephalogram; EMG, submental electromyogram; ECG, electrocardiogram; SUM, weighted sum of the RC and ABD proportional to tidal volume; CO_2, end-tidal CO_2; THERM, thermistor; PULSE, pulse waveform; SaO_2, oxygen saturation percent values; ACT, actimeter; LEOG, REOG, left and right electrooculogram

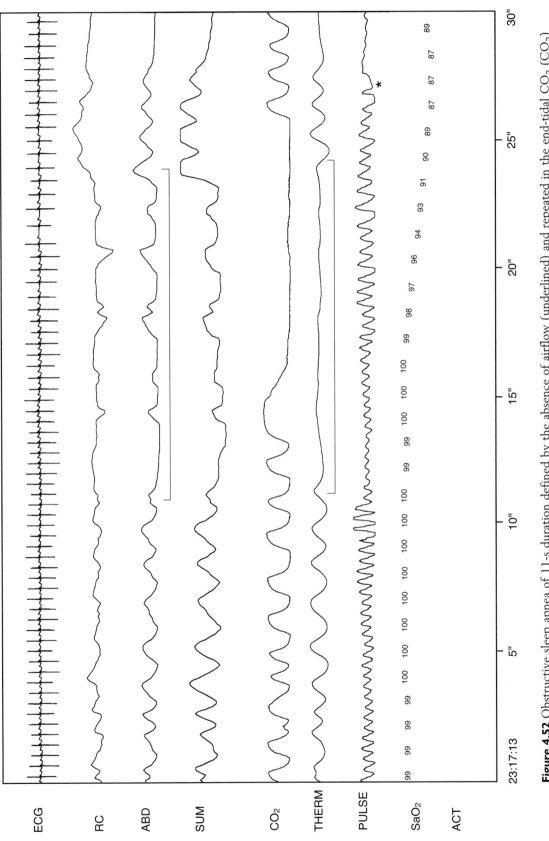

Figure 4.52 Obstructive sleep apnea of 11-s duration defined by the absence of airflow (underlined) and repeated in the end-tidal CO_2 (CO_2) channel after a delay to onset. Out-of-phase rib cage (RC) and abdominal (ABD) breaths that increase in amplitude (underlined) begin within about 3 s after the cessation of airflow. Oxygen saturation (SaO_2) drops to 87% before the pulse signal is lost (*). A brief sinus bradycardia in the electrocardiogram (ECG) can be seen prior to the resumption of airflow. SUM, weighted sum of the RC and ABD proportional to tidal volume; THERM, thermistor; PULSE, pulse waveform; SaO_2, oxygen saturation; ACT, actimeter

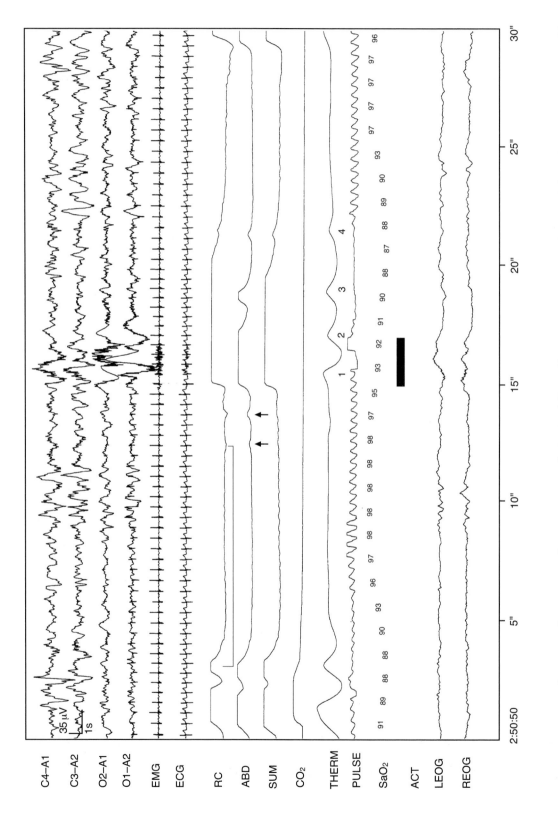

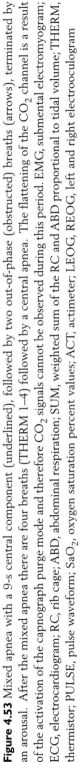

Figure 4.53 Mixed apnea with a 9-s central component (underlined), followed by two out-of-phase (obstructed) breaths (arrows), terminated by an arousal. After the mixed apnea there are four breaths (THERM 1–4) followed by a central apnea. The flattening of the CO_2 channel is a result of the activation of the capnograph purge mode and therefore CO_2 signals cannot be observed during this period. EMG, submental electromyogram; ECG, electrocardiogram; RC, rib cage; ABD, abdominal respiration; SUM, weighted sum of the RC and ABD proportional to tidal volume; THERM, thermistor; PULSE, pulse waveform; SaO_2, oxygen saturation percent values; ACT, actimeter; LEOG, REOG, left and right electrooculogram

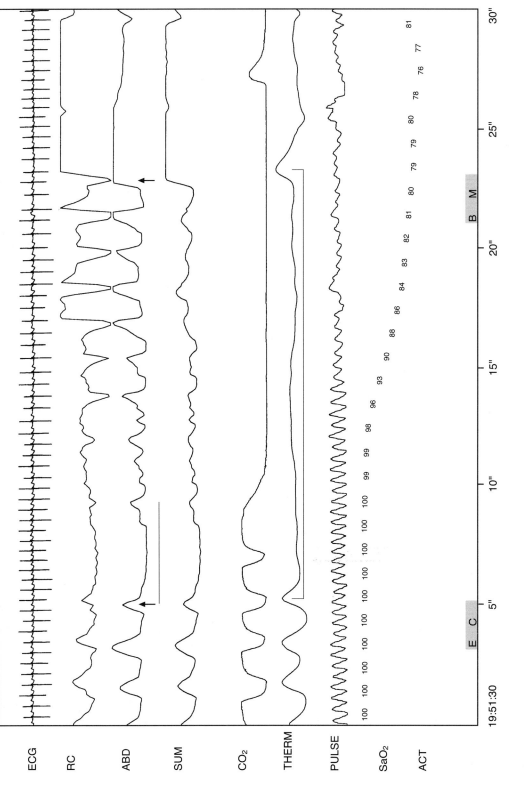

Figure 4.54 Predominantly obstructive mixed apnea (THERM, underlined) and starting and ending at the arrows with a 4-s central period (underlined) followed by a 15-s obstructive component. Note the increasing amplitude of the out-of-phase rib cage (RC) and abdominal (ABD) breaths until they terminate with blocking of the respiratory effort channels. Sinus bradycardia occurs during the obstructed portion along with progressive oxygen desaturation to a low of 76%. The disruption in the pulse signal at about 16 s weakens the validity of the lowest values. ECG, electrocardiogram; SUM, weighted sum of the RC and ABD proportional to tidal volume; CO_2, end-tidal CO_2; THERM, thermistor; PULSE, pulse waveform; SaO_2, oxygen saturation percent values; ACT, actimeter; EC, eyes closed; BM, body movement

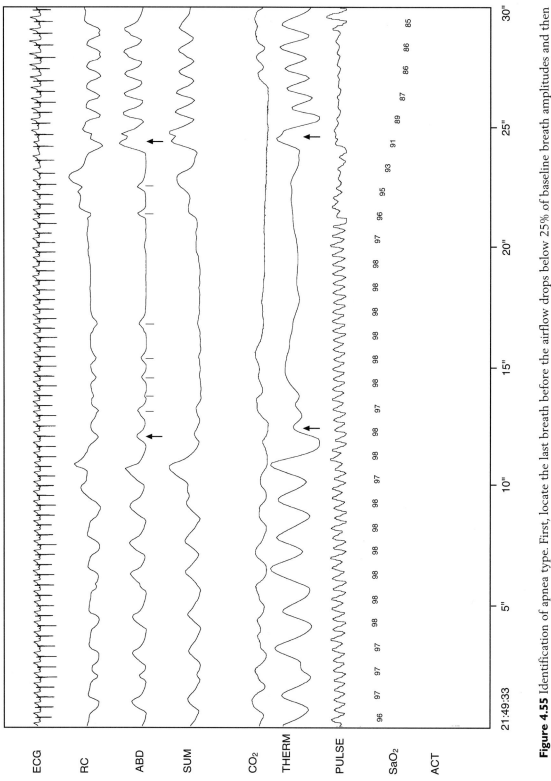

Figure 4.55 Identification of apnea type. First, locate the last breath before the airflow drops below 25% of baseline breath amplitudes and then the next breath above the 25% threshold (arrows). Second, look at the rib cage (RC) and abdominal (ABD) respiration channels during the same time period (arrows) to determine if breaths are present. If yes, as marked by the vertical dashes in this example, this is a central apnea. If not, the out-of-phase breaths would qualify as an obstructed apnea. ECG, electrocardiogram; SUM, weighted sum of the RC and ABD proportional to tidal volume; CO_2, end-tidal CO_2; THERM, thermistor; PULSE, pulse waveform; SaO_2, oxygen saturation percent values; ACT, actimeter

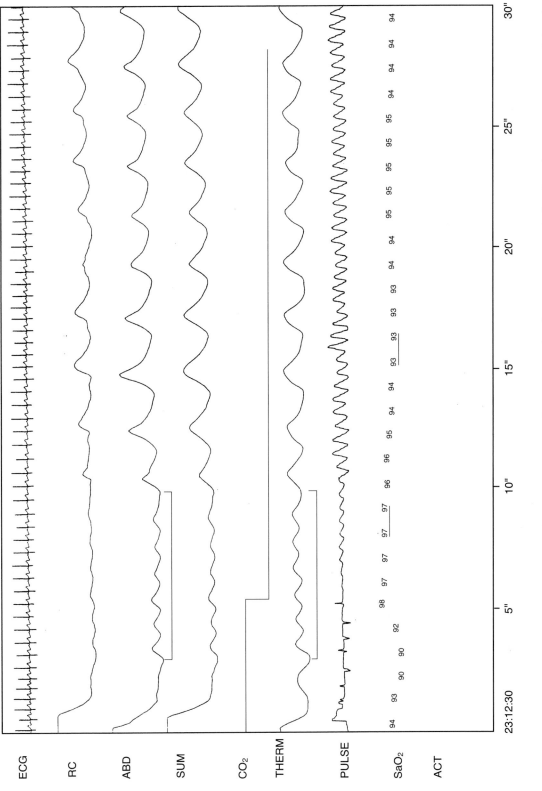

Figure 4.56 Hypopnea. This example reveals a 50% decrease in the presence of airflow (THERM, underlined) and respiratory motion of the rib cage (RC) and abdomen (ABD, underlined) and a 4% decrease in oxygen saturation (SaO_2) (97%–93%, underlined), but it does not meet the ≥10-s duration for scoring. The RC and ABD breaths are perhaps partially out-of-phase, but determining if this is a central or obstructed event will depend on laboratory specific criteria. ECG, electrocardiogram; SUM, weighted sum of the RC and ABD proportional to tidal volume; CO_2, end-tidal CO_2; THERM, thermistor; PULSE, pulse waveform; SaO_2, oxygen saturation percent values; ACT, actimeter

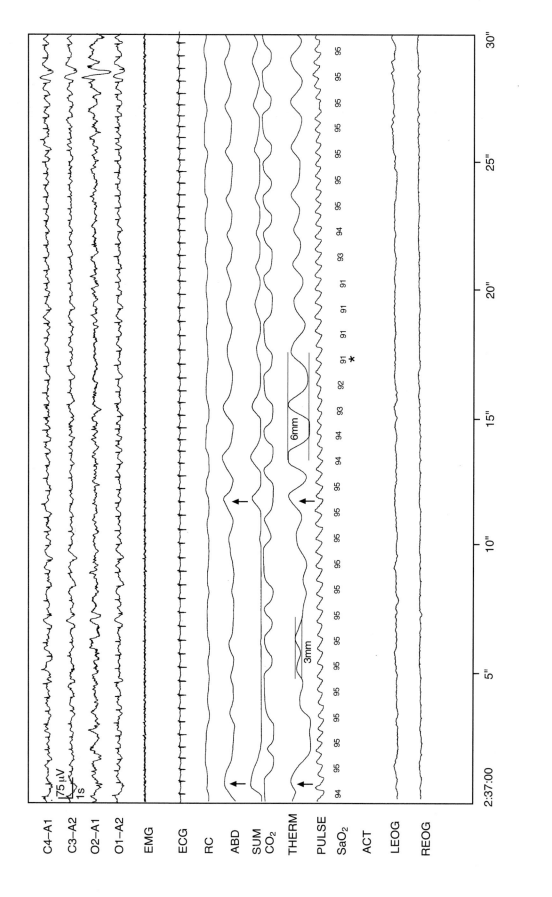

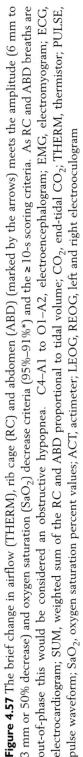

Figure 4.57 The brief change in airflow (THERM), rib cage (RC) and abdomen (ABD) (marked by the arrows) meets the amplitude (6 mm to 3 mm or 50% decrease) and oxygen saturation (SaO_2) decrease criteria (95%–91%*) and the ≥10-s scoring criteria. As RC and ABD breaths are out-of-phase this would be considered an obstructive hypopnea. C4–A1 to O1–A2, electroencephalogram; EMG, electromyogram; ECG, electrocardiogram; SUM, weighted sum of the RC and ABD proportional to tidal volume; CO_2, end-tidal CO_2; THERM, thermistor; PULSE, pulse waveform; SaO_2, oxygen saturation percent values; ACT, actimeter; LEOG, REOG, left and right electrooculogram

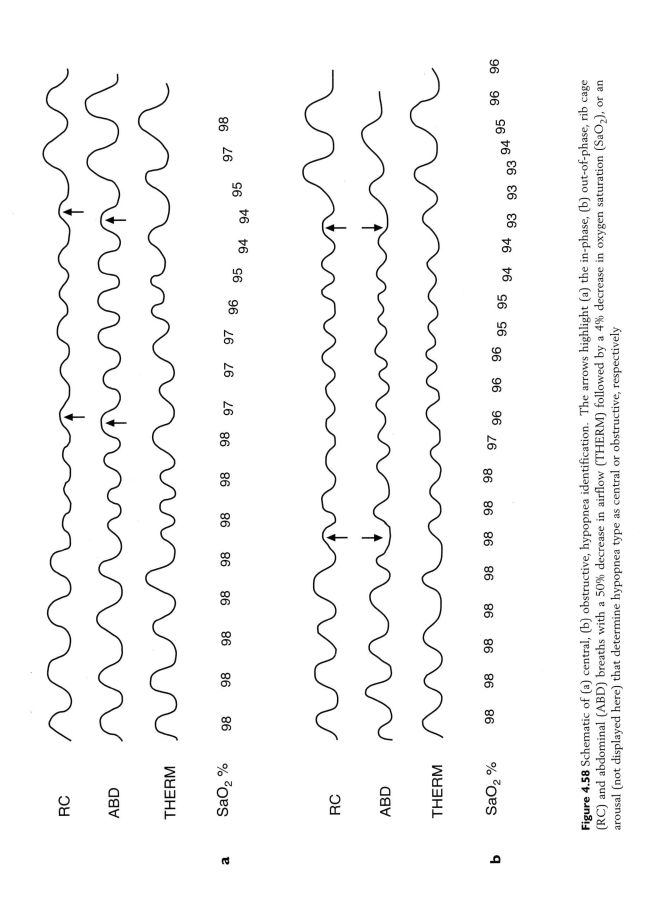

Figure 4.58 Schematic of (a) central, (b) obstructive, hypopnea identification. The arrows highlight (a) the in-phase, (b) out-of-phase, rib cage (RC) and abdominal (ABD) breaths with a 50% decrease in airflow (THERM) followed by a 4% decrease in oxygen saturation (SaO$_2$), or an arousal (not displayed here) that determine hypopnea type as central or obstructive, respectively

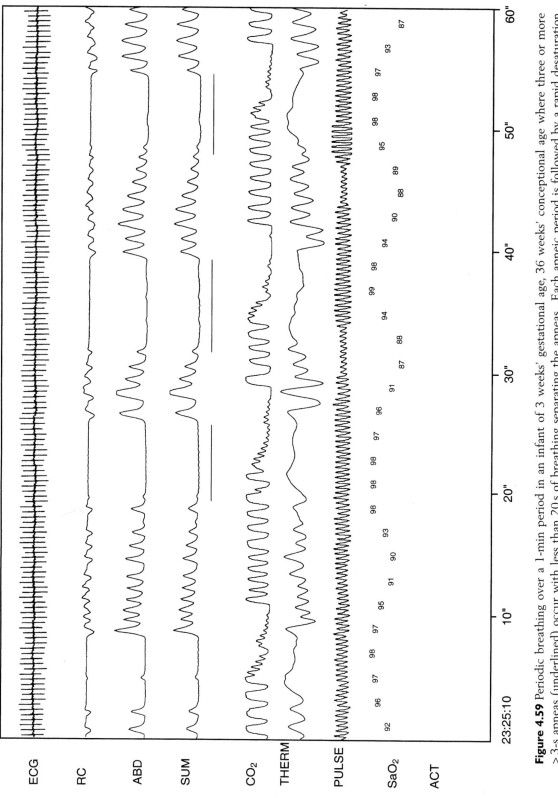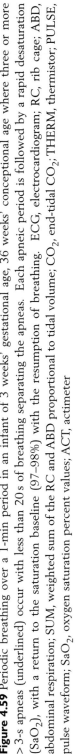

Figure 4.59 Periodic breathing over a 1-min period in an infant of 3 weeks' gestational age, 36 weeks' conceptional age where three or more > 3-s apneas (underlined) occur with less than 20 s of breathing separating the apneas. Each apneic period is followed by a rapid desaturation (SaO_2), with a return to the saturation baseline (97–98%) with the resumption of breathing. ECG, electrocardiogram; RC, rib cage; ABD, abdominal respiration; SUM, weighted sum of the RC and ABD proportional to tidal volume; CO_2, end-tidal CO_2; THERM, thermistor; PULSE, pulse waveform; SaO_2, oxygen saturation percent values; ACT, actimeter

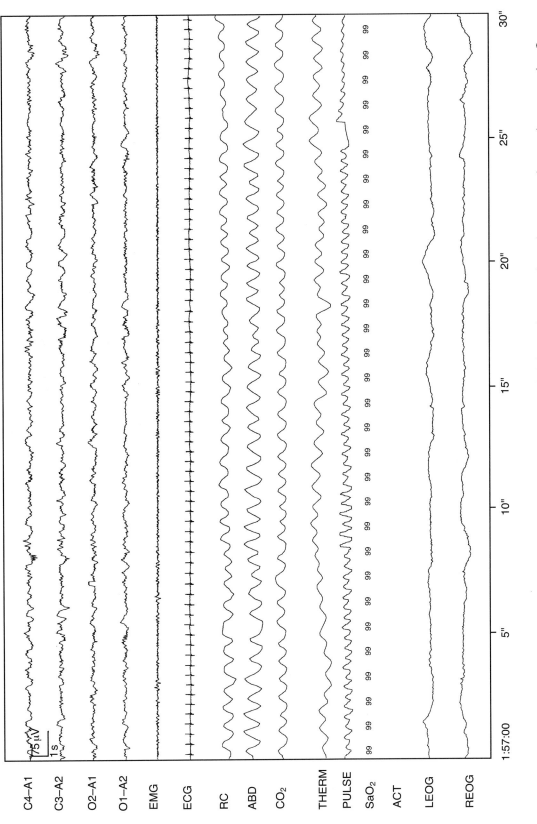

Figure 4.60 Out-of-phase (paradoxical) breathing in the rib cage (RC) and abdominal (ABD) channels in active sleep with continued airflow (THERM) and no oxygen desaturation (SaO_2). This is commonly seen and without a change in airflow amplitude, arousal or desaturation, no event is scored. C4–A1 to O1–A2, electroencephalogram; EMG, electromyogram; ECG, electrocardiogram; SUM, weighted sum of the RC and ABD proportional to tidal volume; CO_2, end-tidal CO_2; THERM, thermistor; PULSE, pulse waveform; SaO_2, oxygen saturation percent values; ACT, actimeter; LEOG, REOG, left and right electrooculogram

Name :_____   MRN: _____   Date: _____

Age: _____   Sex: _____   Study no: _____

Protocol: _____

Referring physician: _____

Indication: _____

Sleep Summary

Lights out: _____

Lights on: _____

Time in bed (min): _____   Wake before sleep (min): _____

Total sleep time (min): _____   Wake during sleep (min): _____

Sleep efficiency: _____   Arousals: _____   Spontaneous: _____   Total QS/NREM _____   AS/REM _____

Latency to sleep: _____   Apnea/hypopnea related: _____

% State   Wake _____   AS _____   QS _____   IS _____

Latency (min)   _____   _____   _____   _____

% Stage   Wake _____   Stg 1 _____   Stg 2 _____   Stg 3 _____   Stg 4 _____   REM _____

Latency (min)   _____   _____   _____   _____   _____   _____

Respiratory Summary

	QS/NREM	Total avg.	Duration (s)	AS/REM	Total avg.	Duration (s)
OSA		_____	_____		_____	_____
Mixed		_____	_____		_____	_____
Central		_____	_____		_____	_____

	Total	QS/NREM	AS/REM		% Total time
Apnea	_____	_____	_____		_____
Hypopnea	_____	_____	_____		_____
Apnea index	_____	_____	_____		_____
A+H index	_____	_____	_____		_____

Oxygen saturation summary   **Cardiac summary**

Wake SaO$_2$: _____   Time below _____ %: _____   Wake HR (bpm) _____

Avg. sleep HR (bpm) _____

PAC _____

PVC _____

	Total	QS/NREM	AS/REM
SaO$_2$ min:	_____	_____	_____
SaO$_2$ mean:	_____	_____	_____

Bodily activity summary

Number of movements: Total _____   QS/NREM _____   AS/REM _____

Movement index: _____

Comments:

Impression:

Signature _____   Date _____

Figure 4.61 Infant polysomnogram report. NREM, non-rapid eye movement; REM, rapid eye movement; AS, active sleep; QS, quiet sleep; IS, indeterminate sleep; OSA, obstructive sleep apnea; avg, average

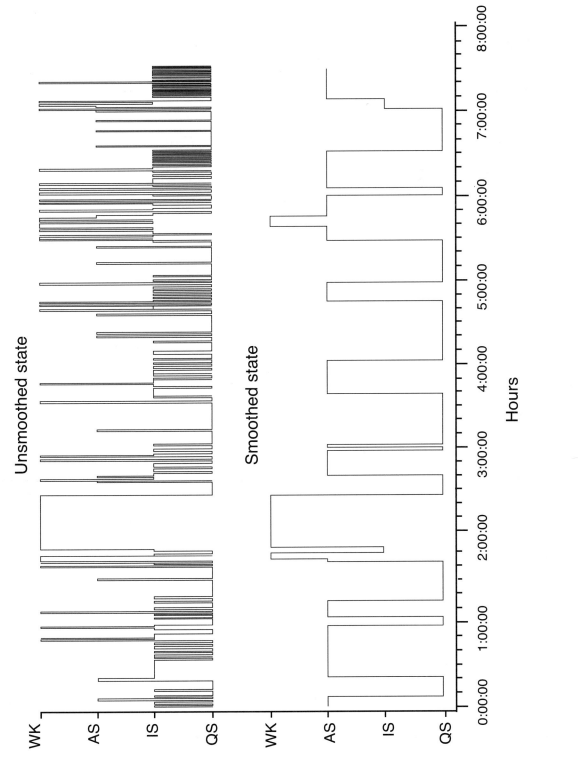

Figure 4.62 Infant nocturnal sleep hypnogram for an 8-h period, illustrating unsmoothed and smoothed representations of sleep state. WK, wake; AS, active sleep; IS, indeterminate sleep; QS, quiet sleep

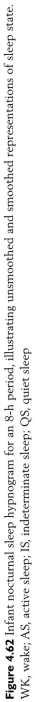

APPENDIX A Caregiver education

Parent(s) and caregivers should receive information on the purpose of the IPSG and what can be expected in the laboratory. A photograph album is a good method for illustrating procedures; questions should be encouraged. Easy-to-read handouts in the appropriate language(s) should be available.

These handouts should contain information about where the IPSG is to be conducted, what the parents need to bring, and when they are expected to bring the baby to the sleep laboratory. Examples of materials used by CHIME follow.

SAMPLE CAREGIVER IPSG EXPLANATION HANDOUT

What is the all-night sleep study?

In order to understand more about how your baby sleeps and how s/he breathes while asleep, an all-night sleep study is conducted to record many different things that occur while your baby sleeps. By placing small sensors on your baby's head, face, chest and foot, we can record brain waves, eye movements, breathing patterns, mouth and nose breathing, heart beats, oxygen levels, movements and body position. These data will be evaluated and results will be forwarded to your baby's doctor. The sensors are placed on the skin with tape and sticky paste and are easily removed when the sleep study is completed. If you wish, you will be able to observe what these recordings look like during the night. The all-night sleep study is a routine, non-invasive procedure.

Upon arrival at the Sleep Lab, sufficient time will be taken so that you and your baby are comfortable in the sleep laboratory. You should be prepared to feed your baby and get him/her ready for bed while the technicians prepare for the recording session. The technicians will explain what they are doing as they prepare your baby for the sleep study and are available to answer any questions.

SAMPLE INSTRUCTIONS TO PARENTS

The all-night sleep study instructions to parents

The all-night sleep study for _____ has been scheduled for 7 pm on _____.

Please bring the following with you:

1. Extra clothes for your baby (i.e. snap-front sleeper)

2. Favorite blanket, sheet, toy, pacifier, etc.

3. A sufficient supply of disposable diapers

4. Enough formula and bottles, if baby is bottle fed

5. Expressed breast milk if mother will not breastfeed

6. Any medications your baby needs

One or both parents should bring _____ to the Sleep Lab at 6:45 pm. The lab is located at the Clinic/Hospital at this address. Parking in the parking lot will be validated. Follow the directional signs to the Sleep Lab. The phone number is _____. A technician will greet you when you arrive.

The longer your baby sleeps, the more valuable information we can obtain from the all-night study. You will be staying at the Sleep Lab until the sleep study is completed in the morning. If there is another sleep room available, you may be able to sleep there during this time. Please be prepared to stay until 7 am.

APPENDIX B Infant polysomnography checklist

The following checklist example is modified from the version used in the CHIME study. A similar document can be made a part of every IPSG record.

IPSG CHECKLIST

This checklist is to be filled out by the PSG technicians during the IPSG recording. **ALL ITEMS SHOULD BE COMPLETED**. Record additional comments if necessary.

1. General information:

_____ Infant's name   _____ ID number

_____/_____/_____ Date of recording

2. Staff information: Who performed IPSG and when were they there?

Name	Staff IN time	Staff OUT time
_____	_____	_____
_____	_____	_____
_____	_____	_____
_____	_____	_____

3. Equipment preparation (Fill in the blank or circle Yes or No): these items can be checked prior to infant arrival.

_____ Software version

Yes   No $EtCO_2$ monitor used? If Yes: Brand and model #:_____

Yes   No   Video monitoring equipment used?

Yes   No   40 W light used?

Yes   No   Crash cart available?

_____ EEG electrode brand?

_____ EMG electrode brand?

_____ EOG electrode brand?

4. Infant preparation:

_____ Infant arrival time

Yes   No   Did parent stay for IPSG?   If Yes: Where did they stay? _____

                                            Who stayed?   _____

Were parents instructed not to intervene?   Yes   No

Yes   No   Is infant using a pacifier?

_____ How was infant clothed and covered for IPSG?

_____ How was infant positioned at start of IPSG?

5. Sensor application (prior to begin study):

Sensors: C3–M2 _____kOhms   Record EEG and EOG impedances

                  C4–M1 _____kOhms   Should be < 5 k

                  O1–M2 _____kOhms   Must be < 10 k

                  O2–M1 _____kOhms

                  _____ # EMG electrodes used? (should be 3)

                  Yes   No   M1+ M2 reference used? (should be Yes)

                  Yes   No   Thermistor used?

                  Yes   No   ECG electrodes applied?

                  Yes No   Actimeter applied to right foot?

                  _____ Respiratory effort sensor type?

Yes No SaO_2 probe attached to left foot?

Yes No   Position sensor on rear of diaper with blue dot facing you?

Yes No $EtCO_2$ monitor used? If Yes,

                Lag time < 1 s?   Yes No

                Was tubing modified?   Yes No

                    If Yes, how: _____

6. Before starting:

_____   Time recorder turned on?

Yes   No   Filters set correctly?

Yes   No $EtCO_2$ monitor turned on and working properly?

Yes   No   Signal qualities good? (If No, make an attempt to fix before calibration)

_____   Time calibration started?

Yes   No   1 minute calibration completed?

_____   Time 'Begin study' was entered in Comments?

7. During IPSG recording:

Infant behavior codes should be entered directly into the computer.

ALL interventions should also be entered into the computer and recorded in detail below:

Start time   Stop time   Description *(i.e. infant feeding, diaper change, technical adjustments, etc.):*

_____   _____   _____

_____   _____   _____

_____   _____   _____

_____   _____   _____

_____   _____   _____

_____	_____	_____
_____	_____	_____
_____	_____	_____
_____	_____	_____
_____	_____	_____

Record the room temperature: @21.00:_____ °C

@01.30:_____ °C

@04.00:_____ °C

8. Termination of recording (Note: PSG should continue for a MINIMUM of 8 hours after time 'Begin study' was entered):

Recheck impedances: C3–M2_____kOhms

C4–M1_____kOhms

O1–M2_____kOhms

O2–M1_____kOhms

Yes   No   Enter 'End study' in Comments?

_____   Time 'End study' was entered in Comments?

Yes   No   1 minute End calibration performed?

_____   Time end calibration was started?

_____   Time data acquisition stopped?

_____   Time computer powered off?

9. Technician comments (i.e. signal quality, clinical observations, etc.). Attach additional pages if necessary:

10. PSG documentation and data storage/backup:

Yes   No   Data copied to storage media?   File No:_____

APPENDIX C Modification of the International 10–20 system measurements for infant polysomnography

Seven EEG electrodes (C3, C4, O1, O2, M1, M2, Ground) will be placed on the scalp and held in place with electrode paste.

Modified directions for locating the International 10–20 system sites for these electrodes follow:

- Even numbers refer to the right side of the head; odd numbers to the left (Z is the midline)

- Use a flexible, disposable/washable centimeter measuring tape and

- Place the zero (0) end of the tape on the nasion (depression between the nose and forehead) and direct the tape to the back of the head. Read off the cm at the inion (the protuberance at the back of the head)

- With the tape still held in place, locate the halfway point of your nasion–inion distance. For example, if the nasion–inion distance is 25 cm, 12.5 is the midpoint. Mark this point (CZ)

- Leaving the tape in place, measure up 10% from the nasion (2.5 cm in this example). This is the FPZ site on the forehead midline. Locate ground electrode about 30% of the distance from the nasion to the hairline at this midline point

- Repeat this process from the inion: 10% up on the midline is OZ

- Remove the tape and place one end on the preauricular point (the depression in front of the ear) and direct the tape across the head through the CZ mark to the other preauricular point. Note the distance in cm

- With the tape in place find the point that is half the 'ear to ear' distance and mark the intersection with your nasion–inion CZ mark

- With the tape still in place, measure up 10% from the preauricular point on each side of the head; mark this point, then measure an additional 20%; this is C3 on the left side and C4 on the right side

- Measure the circumference of the head by placing the tape along the 10% markings all the way around. Note half the distance and then calculate 10% of this distance

- Mark 10% to the left and right of FPZ; these points are FP1 and FP2. Direct the tape through FP1 back to the 10% marks on the left side of the inion at the circumference line. Mark the intersection. This intersection is O1. Repeat this process on the right side from FP2 to locate O2

- M1 and M2 are the left and right mastoids, respectively. Palpate the bone behind the ear and avoid any blood vessels to reduce ECG artifact

APPENDIX D Documentation

CAREGIVING, INTERVENTIONS AND INFANT BEHAVIORS

Information on technical decisions and environmental conditions can be entered on a form or checklist such as that in Appendix B. Documentation of caregiving, interventions and infant behaviors must be entered as they occur on the paper tracing or computer comments fields. Some computers have limited space and time to enter comments and entries may stray from the point of occurrence if they are protracted. Therefore, it is very useful to have a set of standardized abbreviations to identify the many activities that take place during a nocturnal IPSG (see Behavior coding section that follows).

The CHIME study discriminated between caregiver actions and technician/parent interventions as follows: all caregiving was denoted by the word, 'BEGIN' at the point the caregiving begins, then the caregiving was described, then the word 'END' was entered when it was completed. Caregiving procedures are those that generally involve the infant being in the awake state. Examples include:

- Infant feedings: what, how long, amount, burping periods, etc.

- Diaper changes

- Comforting, patting, rocking

Other interventions are identified by 'IN' when the person enters the infant's room, describe the intervention, then enter 'OUT'.

These are interventions that do not necessarily awaken the infant. Examples include:

- Nurse/parent/technician entering the sleep room

- Nurse/parent/technician touching the infant

- Removal or addition of blankets

- Re-application of sensors, i.e. $EtCO_2$, ECG, SaO_2

- Responses to alarms

- Emergency procedures

Behavior coding

Abbreviations	Definition	Description
Awake vs. asleep periods		
EO	eyes open	indicates that the infant is awake
EC	eyes closed	indicates that the infant is asleep*
	* If infant is alseep and no behaviors are noted for 5 minutes, enter EC	
Interventions		
IN	person IN infant's room	enter IN, then describe the intervention then enter OUT
OUT	person OUT of infant's room	
Caregiving		
BEGIN	beginning of caregiving period	enter BEGIN, describe the caregiving, then enter END
END	end of caregiving period	
Body movements		
BM	body movements	use BM to describe any of the body movements listed below:
	• stretching	slow, extending movement of trunk or hand or extremities
	• rolling over	change in position between lateral, supine or prone
	• jerky movement	accelerated, quick movement involving one or more extremities
	• twitching	repetitive, sudden, quick jerky motion
	• writhing	twisting or turning movements, squirming, contorting
	• limb movements	movement of one or more extremities
STR	startle	sudden, unexpected movement, usually involving all extremities
FM	facial movements	use FM to describe movements involving the face and mouth:
	• smiling	joyful facial expression
	• grimacing	discontented facial expression
	• yawning	wide, open mouth, with prolonged inhalation
MO	mouthing	repetitive opening and closing of the mouth
SUCK	sucking	periodic sucking movements of mouth and lips
SIGH	sigh	long, deep audible exhalation
Pacifier use		
BPAC	begin pacifier	the infant has begun using a pacifier
EPAC	end pacifier	the infant has ended the use of a pacifier
Vocalizations		
BCRY	begin cry	beginning of a crying period
ECRY	end cry	end of a crying period
VOC	other vocalizations	sounds produced by the infant, including those listed below:
	• whimpers	low, whining, broken cry sounds
	• babbling	incoherent vocal sounds
	• grunting	short, deep, hoarse sounds
	• hiccough	sharp, quick sound caused by involuntary contraction of diaphragm

APPENDIX E Quality review

Quality review, i.e. assessment of the technical quality of the IPSG, can provide important, written documentation regarding sleep laboratory performance and promote continued performance improvement. Feedback to technicians and managers can serve as a vehicle for discussion and monitoring of quality improvement. The CHIME study prepared a special form for this purpose and determined which aspects of the IPSG would be essential to data required for analysis. A trained reviewer scanned each IPSG, completed the Quality Review Form and sent a copy to the sleep laboratory. The following paragraphs summarize the contents of this particular form.

Header section Demographics regarding the infant, date of IPSG, name of reviewer, date of review, etc.

Signal quality Summarizes each channel of data. A subjective determination is made as to whether the signals are of sufficient quality to be used for scoring purposes. In general, the quality of the signal must be adequate for at least two-thirds (66%) of the night. Channels may be highlighted to focus on those most important to sleep state, respiratory scoring as appropriate. If a signal is deemed unscorable for the majority of the night, a comment is made as to the reason for the signal being unscorable.

Annotations Awake periods must be clearly marked. Movements should be clearly annotated.

Filter setting Accuracy should be verified and discrepancies highlighted.

Calibrations EEG and EMG calibrations are checked for accuracy and discrepancies highlighted.

Data stored Verify that the entire recording period was stored on back-up media as appropriate.

Overall comments Enter general summary comments.

APPENDIX F Apnea/hypopnea measurement

CHIME GUIDELINES FOR MEASURING APNEA AND HYPOPNEA ON PAPER OR USING COMPUTER-ASSISTED MEASUREMENT TOOLS

General guidelines

- Determine durations of respiratory disturbances that will be considered as measurable events

- Determine if you will measure an event that occurs during sleep, even if the epoch is scored as wakefulness

- If you have a computerized system that 'automatically' scores events according to preset filters, you will need to review all epochs to verify the accuracy of these detected events and rescore if necessary

- Select the channels that will constitute the montage for respiratory event scoring. CHIME used ECG, rib cage, abdomen, sum, CO_2, thermistor (nasal/oral airflow), pulse waveform, oxygen saturation and actimeter

Apnea rules

- The primary channel to observe is airflow for the initial determination of absence or reduction of airflow. The most artifact resistant channel is the CO_2; therefore, this channel should be used to identify the breaths preceding and following the airflow cessation (or reduction)

- Measure apnea duration from the end of inspiration to the end of the next inspiration ('peak to peak')

- If there is a discrepancy between CO_2 duration and thermistor duration, use the channel that gives the shortest apnea duration for determining the beginning and end point of the apnea

- Consult the abdominal channel and verify whether there was a simultaneous cessation in respiratory movements. If the answer is yes, the apnea can be considered central. If there are obstructed breaths during this period, the event will be classified as obstructive or mixed according to your laboratory rules

Other apnea measurement considerations

- Cardiogenic artifacts often can be observed in the CO_2 or thermistor channels. In order not to confuse these with breaths, check the ECG frequency and ignore those waves that coincide with the heartbeats or SaO_2 pulse waveform. The thermistor may provide a clue to the first real breath or resumption of breathing after an apnea

- When CO_2 is recorded there may be a delay of 1 s (sometimes more) between changes in the CO_2 waveform and other respiratory signals. The term 'simultaneous' presupposes that any delay be discounted

- In some cases, only a thermistor channel may be available. This can be used as an alternative to CO_2. If both are in use, the beginning and end of an apnea must be timed on the same channel

- If the preceding or subsequent breath is broad, without a peak, identify the middle of that breath as the peak. If breaths are more easily identified on the thermistor channel, time the apnea using this channel

- The first breath or few breaths following a central apnea may be paradoxical with reduced airflow. However, the central apnea terminates at the *first* effort, even if the breath is out-of-phase

- The first breath following a central apnea may be paradoxical without airflow (obstructed breath) yet this obstructed component may not last the duration necessary to meet the criteria for mixed apnea. The termination of central apnea is timed with the return of respiratory efforts

- When CO_2 and thermistor are recorded, use the channel that gives you the shortest apnea duration

Hypopnea rules

- View a montage that includes ECG, rib cage and abdominal movements (sum (VT) if using RIP), CO_2, thermistor, pulse waveform, SaO_2 and actimeter

- If you have a computerized system, set the filters to automatically identify drops of thermistor amplitude of 50% or more. Do not ignore eligible events not identified by the computer. If measuring the drop manually, compare the possible event amplitude to the amplitude of baseline/normal breaths

- Examine each flagged/possible hypopnea. Verify the 4% drop in SaO_2. In order to accept the validity of the SaO_2 signal, there should be at least three acceptable pulse waves. If artifact prevails, this latter criterion is not fulfilled and the SaO_2 cannot be used to accept or reject the hypopnea. The SaO_2 drop should occur either during the hypopneic event or within seconds after the termination of this event

- Check if a scorable arousal is contingent on this event. An arousal is contingent if it occurs during or within 5 s after the termination of the hypopneic event. If at least one of the two criteria is not fulfilled, the possible event cannot be scored as a hypopnea

- The beginning of a hypopneic event is defined by the peak of the last 'full' breath, i.e. the breath before the amplitude dropped by 50%. The termination of an hypopneic event is defined as the peak of the first breath with an amplitude at least equal to the last full breath before the 50% drop

- Consult the ribcage and abdominal channels to determine if it is central or obstructive hypopnea. If breaths in these two channels are in-phase, it is a central hypopnea. If these two channels are not in-phase, it is an obstructive hypopnea

Other consideration

- It is possible that movements prevent accurate identification of central and especially obstructive hypopnea. Check sleep states to determine if the infant was awake. If so, do not score the event. If the infant was asleep, indicate that this hypopnea was 'uninterpretable'

APPENDIX G Elimination of spurious and artifactual signals

ELIMINATION OF SPURIOUS OXIMETRY DATA

The pulse waveform indicates the quality of the oximeter data. A rounded, upgoing signal should be present for each QRS complex on the ECG, although the pulse waveform will be slightly delayed. Any significant decrease in amplitude may indicate a concomitant decrease in SaO_2 reliability. When the pulse signal identifies unreliable data, the SaO_2 signal must be eliminated for that segment and 5 s beyond, i.e. the length of the oximeter averaging window.

ELIMINATION OF SPURIOUS END-TIDAL CO_2 DATA

When the end-tidal CO_2 signal becomes artifactual, it should be removed from calculations for the overnight study. The CO_2 signal is subject to artifact, usually due to displacement or plugging of the nasal catheter leading to falsely low values. Accurate CO_2 signals are characterized by a smooth, end-expiratory plateau, with small variations in amplitude from breath to breath. With rapid respiratory rates, a smooth peak is sometimes observed rather than a plateau. End-tidal CO_2 readings should be considered artifactual under the following circumstances:

- If the nasal/oral thermistor signal shows stable baseline flow, but the CO_2 amplitude is reduced from baseline by one-third or more, then that portion of the CO_2 should be considered artifact, and the data should not be included in summary calculations

- If the technician notes that the catheter has been displaced or plugged and replaces the catheter, the affected data preceding the catheter replacement should be discarded

- If the signal is disrupted from movement secondary to catheter displacement and the signal spontaneously returns to the previous baseline, the affected data should be removed. Obstructive sleep apnea can occur in association with movement, so these data should be evaluated carefully before they are removed from the calculations

CARDIAC SIGNALS

- If the heart rate drops precipitously due to a loose electrode or an artifact for at least three beats, remove the signal for scoring results

Glossary

Accelerometer

A sensor that measures acceleration due to gravity changes that can be used to monitor position or movement, i.e. a transducer that converts body motion into an electrical signal.

Activity (electroencephalogram (EEG))

An EEG wave or sequence of waves classified by frequency, i.e. alpha activity 8–13 Hz.

Active sleep state

The state of infant sleep prior to about 3 months' adjusted age considered equivalent to Stage REM.

Adjusted age

Chronological age expressed as the age since birth calculated from the time when the infant would have been at term; for example, 3 months' adjusted age in a baby born at 35 weeks' GA would count the 3 months starting at 40 weeks or when the baby reached 'term'.

Airflow

Movement of air from the nose and/or mouth detected by inspired/expired gases (such as carbon dioxide (CO_2)) or temperature.

Alpha EEG frequency band (alpha rhythm)

Brain waves that cycle between 8 and 13 times/s in children and adults, characteristic of the relaxed awake state with eyes closed. In infants, alpha may occur but it is not a hallmark of the awake state; frequencies may be slower in infants (< 8 Hz) until about 7–8 years of age. The amplitude tends to be highest in the parietal or occipital regions.

Amplitude

The trough–peak or peak–trough distance of a wave compared to a standard signal in μV or mV. The maximum voltage between two points.

Analog signals

Voltages that vary in time in proportion to the physiological quantity they represent.

Analog-to-digital conversion

Process of changing analog signals to a numerical form that can be accepted by digital computers. The numerical format represents the value of the signal at predetermined, uniformly spaced intervals of time.

Apnea

'Absence' of breath, generally defined by absence of airflow at nose and mouth. In polysomnography, apnea generally refers to events of ≥ 10-s duration, but < 10 s may be considered significant in children.

Arousal (EEG arousal)

Transient, abrupt changes in EEG frequency reflecting a change from deep to lighter sleep or sleep to wake. Arousal may be associated with increases in tonic electromyogram (EMG), heart rate and body movements.

Asystole

No detectable cardiac activity on the electro-cardiogram (ECG).

Atrial

Activity arising in the atria of the heart.

Atrioventricular block (AVB)

Delay of the impulse within the AV node, resulting in a longer than normal pause before stimulation of the ventrical, i.e. a pause between the P-wave and the QRS or a P without the following QRS.

Autonomic nervous system

The part of the nervous system that is not subject to voluntary control but that regulates life-preserving functions such as heart rate and respiration.

Awake state (stage)

A non-sleep state characterized by EEG similar to active sleep (beta/theta), an increase in tonic EMG, voluntary rapid eye movements and eye blinks in conjunction with the presence of an alert state or awareness of the environment. In infants and young children, behavioral observation of eyes open, alert look, crying or feeding are important for the confirmation of the awake state.

Band pass filter

Filter that passes a range of frequencies while rejecting those above or below the specified range.

Beta EEG frequency band

Brain waves that cycle at 13–35 Hz; often associated with alert wakefulness, accompanied by high/elevated tonic EMG. This rhythm may be drug-induced.

Bioelectric signals

Electrical signals that appear in the body and on its surface.

Bioelectrical potential

A single potential generated by neural or muscle tissue as a discrete event with measurable variables (size, configuration, etc.).

Biopotential electrode

Sensors that detect changes in bioelectric signals in the body to signals that can be conducted through wires connected to a recording device.

Bipolar derivation

Where two scalp electrodes are connected to make up the derivation.

Blocking

Loss of the recorded signal at the highest or lowest edge of the recording range due to sensitivity or gain setting that is too high or the signal is too large due to movement.

Bradycardia

Heart rate below the expected limits for age, sleep/wake state and activity/status.

Burst

Distinct, abrupt short-lasting change in activity with a difference in amplitude, frequency or waveform.

Canthus

Points where upper and lower eyelids meet, i.e. outer canthus.

Cardiac arrhythmia (dysrhythmia)

Disturbance of impulse formation or conduction or a combination of the two. Arrhythmias generally are separated into two groups: those that originate in the sinus node or in the atrioventricular (AV) node.

Cardiorespiratory monitoring

Physiological monitoring of the heart and respiration; the latter may include both airflow and respiratory effort but often only effort as in impedance recordings on home apnea monitors.

Cardiotachometer

A specialized recording device that converts the ECG R–R interval into beats per minute.

Central apnea

A cessation in airflow and respiratory muscles caused when respiratory control centers fail to activate respiratory movement.

Central nervous system

The brain and spinal cord.

Conceptional age (CA)

Age from conception in weeks.

Continuous EEG waveforms

Continuously varying potentials that persist over long periods, usually sinusoidal in shape.

Cycle

Rhythmic fluctuation, as in a brain wave or respiratory inspiration/expiration, that includes the activity from one maximum or one minimum to the next.

Delta EEG frequency band (delta rhythm)

Brain waves of less than 4 Hz. In adults, the criteria for delta waves are a minimum amplitude of 75 μV and 0.5-s duration (2 Hz) or less. In infants and children, delta wave amplitudes may exceed 50 μV and amplitude increases with age.

Delta-brush EEG waveform pattern

Moderate to high amplitude delta waves with superimposed 8–20 Hz activity in rolandic, temporal and occipital brain areas.

Derivation

The set of connected electrodes recorded as one output signal, e.g. C3–A2 or C3–A1+A2.

Diastole

The time period when the heart is in a state of relaxation and fills with blood.

Digastric muscle

One of the suprahyoid group of muscles with the insertion at the lower border of the mandible near the midline.

Diurnal

Daytime-related.

EEG spikes

A transient clearly distinguished from background activity, 20–< 70 ms, main component is negative and very pointed.

Electrocardiogram (ECG)

Graphic/recorded display of the electrical pulses generated by actions of the heart. Usually referred to by letters (P, Q, R, S, T, U) that represent the various components.

Electroencephalogram (EEG)

Signal detected on the surface of the scalp produced by ensemble brain activity and displayed on a recording instrument. The EEG reflects changes in voltage and frequency of brain waves.

Electroencephalograph

Instrument used to amplify and record the EEG signals.

Electromyogram (EMG)

A recording of electrical activity from the muscles; in sleep recordings, EMG is most often recorded from the digastric or submental muscles. This 'chin' EMG combined with other parameters such as EEG and EOG in children and adults is used to classify sleep states and stages.

Electrooculogram (EOG)

Electrical signal detected on the skin surface in the vicinity of the eyes that is produced by the electrical properties of each eye and electrical changes due to eye movements, displayed on a recording instrument.

Epoch

Sleep state or stage scoring unit time during the polysomnogram, typically 20, 30 or 60 s.

Filter

Electronic circuit with a gain or attenuation factor that favors certain frequencies (pass frequencies) over other unfavored frequencies (reject frequencies).

Frequency range

Range with most of a signal's energy, e.g. in the EEG 0.5–35 Hz.

Gain

The gain of an amplifier is the unit required to increase the amplitude of the signal by a factor greater than one.

Gastroesophageal reflux (GER)

Acidity in the esophagus related to discomfort, regurgitation and possibly apneic events. GER is measured with a miniature pH sensor placed in the esophagus in conjunction with a surface skin electrode.

Gestational age (GA)

Age from conception (defined by last normal menstrual period) to birth, expressed in weeks.

Heart rate

Rate at which the heart beats, expressed as beats per minute (bpm).

Hemoglobin oxygen saturation

Level of oxygen content in the hemoglobin of the blood.

Hertz (Hz)

Term defining a unit of frequency and synonymous with cycles per second (cps). Hz is the preferred term.

High-pass filter

Filter that allows signal components at frequencies above a prescribed value to be passed while those below the cut-off frequency are rejected.

Hypercapnia

Elevated CO_2 in the blood.

Hypopnea

A shallow breathing period (airflow below 50% of baseline) during sleep, associated with a decrease in blood oxygen saturation and/or arousal.

Idiopathic apparent life-threatening event (ALTE) of infancy

An event characterized by change in tone (limpness, stiffness) and color (pallor, cyanosis) with difficulty or absent breathing that requires significant intervention for resolution.

Impedance

Source impedance in time-varying or alternating current (AC) systems associated with biopotential electrodes and most electronic devices. Impedance is a measure of how well the electrode is connected to a biological host as well as how well the electrode is functioning.

Indeterminate sleep state

Infant sleep state that does not meet either quiet or active sleep criteria.

Inductance plethysmography

Inductance refers to the electrical properties of a loop of wire that changes proportionately to measures within the loop. Two loops are necessary to determine changes in the cross-sectional area of, for example, the chest and abdomen, yielding a signal that is proportional to tidal volume.

International 10–20 system

Standardized system of scalp measurement and surface electrode placements used in electro-encephalography and PSG.

K-complex

The combination of a sharp, negative EEG wave directly followed by a high-voltage slow wave at the vertex and frequently associated with a sleep spindle. The complex must be at least 0.5-s duration. The waves may be seen in a rudimentary form in infancy and have more adult characteristics by 7–8 months of age. K-complexes occur spontaneously in quiet or NREM sleep but also can be evoked by external stimuli. They may reflect brief periods of arousal.

Low-pass filter

Filter that allows signal components at frequencies below a prescribed value to be passed and those higher to be rejected. Synonym: high-frequency filter.

Mastoid process

The projection of the petrous portion of the bone behind the ear.

Mercury strain gauge (Hg strain gauge)

An electrical device that produces a signal related to changes in length. This device is often a thin tube filled with mercury. Electrical resistance variation is proportional to the changes in tube length as the tube is stretched and released, e.g. during chest expansion during respiration.

Methylxanthine

A drug derived from the purine derivative xanthine (caffeine, theophylline).

Mixed EEG waveform pattern

Combination of high-voltage EEG slow waves and fast-frequency low-voltage EEG waves without any specific patterning.

Monopolar (referential)

Derivation where an active electrode is referenced to a non-active site such as the ear lobe or mastoid process.

Montage

A specific arrangement by which transducers and/or electrode derivations are displayed simultaneously in the PSG.

Motion artifact

Interference caused by electrode movement that creates an electrical signal of non-biological origin.

Nocturnal sleep

The typical 'night-time' sleep period.

Noise

Any signal or random process that is not the desired signal.

Notch or band reject filter

Filter that rejects a range of frequencies while allowing other frequencies to pass. Notch filters have a very narrow range, e.g. 60 Hz or 50 Hz, often used to reject interference from power mains. If the biological signal contains those frequencies, the output signal may be somewhat distorted.

NREM sleep stages

The sleep periods that are not REM sleep, i.e. non-REM or NREM, comprised of Stages 1–4. These stages can be identified after 3–6 months of adjusted age.

Nyquist criteria

Sampling at least twice the highest expected signal frequency remaining after filtering.

Obstructive sleep apnea

Apneic period with cessation of airflow but continued respiratory effort.

Offset

Process of adding or subtracting a fixed voltage to a signal to move it up or down on the display recording to reduce or eliminate signal blocking.

Out-of-phase breaths

Rib cage–abdominal asynchrony.

Paroxysmal atrial tachycardia (PAT)

Sudden irritable atrial firing producing rapid heart rate, P-waves that look different from SA node-generated waves, followed by normal-appearing QRST cycle.

Phasic EMG

Bursts of muscle activity superimposed on baseline tonic EMG.

Plethysmography

A measurement that determines changes in size or volume.

Pneumogram

Cardiorespiratory recording.

Polarity

Sign of potential difference between electrodes.

Polysomnography/polysomnogram (PSG)

The simultaneous recording of physiological parameters during sleep that must include those for scoring of sleep states or stages (EEG, EOG, EMG). This term also includes the analysis and interpretation of these multiple parameters.

Post-term

Age at birth beyond 42 weeks' CA or, for example, a baby born at term (38–42 weeks' GA) who is now 2 months old may be described as 2 months post-term.

P–R interval

Distance from the beginning of the P-wave to the point where the QRS complex begins. A P–R interval > 0.2 s is referred to as first-degree AV block.

Premature atrial contraction (PAC)

Occurrence of an abnormal P-wave earlier than expected; pacing is reset one cycle length from the premature beat.

Premature ventricular contraction (PVC)

Originating suddenly in a ventricular generating system producing a very large ventricular complex on the ECG. The PVC occurs early in the cycle followed by a compensatory pause not caused by a resetting of the SA node.

Pre-term birth

Gestational age at birth precedes 38 weeks.

Prolonged Q–T interval

The Q–T interval represents the duration of ventricular systole, from the beginning of the QRS to the end of the T-wave. Prolonged Q–T interval is greater than one-half of the R–R interval at a normal heart rate.

Pulse oximeter

Device for non-invasive measurement of oxygen in peripheral tissues by passing light of two different wavelengths through, for example, a finger, hand, toe or foot.

Quiet sleep state

Infant sleep state when Stages 1–4 cannot be determined.

Rapid eye movement(s) (REMs)

Synchronous, abrupt, oppositional deflections of recorded eye movements.

REM sleep stage

Sleep stage associated with increased brain activity and metabolism and dreaming. The EEG has low-voltage mixed-frequency brain waves. Spontaneous REMs occur but other muscle activity is suppressed.

Resistance

Source impedance in direct current (DC) systems.

Respiratory effort

Another term for respiratory muscle activity.

Respiratory pause

A brief period (generally $\leq$3-s duration) after the expiratory phase where no respiratory airflow or effort is observed.

Respiratory sinus arrhythmia (RSA)

A normal physiological variation in SA node pacing rate in association with respiration, shown as a minimal increase in heart rate with inspiration and a minimal decrease with expiration.

Rhythm

The pace or frequency at which physiological impulses/signals occur, as in EEG waveforms or heart rate.

Rolling or slow eye movements

This type of eye movement is characteristic of the onset of Stage 1 sleep.

R–R interval

The time period between one ECG R-wave peak and the next R-wave peak.

Sampling theorem

The sampling rate of a signal must be at least twice the highest frequency component of the signal to fully represent its analog counterpart (Nyquist criteria).

Saturation

Amplifier gain is too high for the signal being processed, resulting in signal truncation or blocking on the output recording.

Saw-tooth EEG waves

A notched-appearing waveform, usually in bursts during REM sleep.

Sensor

Interface between the physiological signal and measuring/recording instrument that converts the physiological variable to an electrical signal that can be processed by the instrument.

Sharp EEG waves

A wave of 70–200 ms that stands out from the background, pointed, but less so than a spike.

Signal-to-noise ratio

Ratio of signal amplitude, energy or power to the noise amplitude, energy or power, usually presented as a logarithmic scale.

Silver/silver chloride (Ag/AgCl) electrode

Non-polarizing electrode that minimizes motion artifact and noise by having a silver chloride surface.

Sinus rhythm

Rhythm generated in the SA node that paces the heart. In a normal sinus rhythm, a constant cycle duration is maintained.

Sinusoid/sinusoidal waves

Term for waves resembling sine waves.

Sleep architecture

The quiet sleep–active sleep (NREM–REM sleep) states and cycles often depicted quantitatively in the form of a histogram (somnogram).

Sleep spindles

Brief, rhythmic bursts of EEG waves in the 11–15 Hz range, generally of highest amplitude in the central region of the head. Sleep spindles are one of the identifying features of Stage 2 sleep.

Sleep state

Sleep period with specifically defined characteristics in infants < 3 months CA.

Sleep state (stage) smoothing

Process of extending the definition of sleep state or stages over more than one epoch in order to decrease the frequency of transient, discrepant states.

Sleep study

Recording of cardiorespiratory (or other) physiological variables during sleep without recording those that define sleep *per se*.

Source impedance

The amount of interference encountered by an electrical current (other than a superconductor) that limits the amount of current that can flow for a particular driving force.

Spontaneous arousal

An arousal without any discernible stimulus.

Stage 1 sleep

Relatively low-voltage mixed-frequency EEG (alpha < 50% of the epoch). Occurs at sleep onset and after arousal from other sleep stages. May contain EEG vertex sharp waves, slow rolling eye movements, but no sleep spindles, K-complexes or REMs.

Stage 2 sleep

NREM sleep stage with < 20% delta waves.

Stage 3 sleep

NREM sleep stage with ≥ 20 but ≤ 50% delta waves.

Stage 4 sleep

NREM sleep stage with > 50% delta waves. Stages 3 and 4 often are combined and have been referred to as 'slow wave sleep'. Stage 4, or arousal from Stage 4, is associated with sleepwalking, sleep terrors and confusional arousal.

Sudden infant death syndrome (SIDS)

Diagnosis assigned to the cause of death in infants under 1 year of age when all other causes have been ruled out.

Synchronous breathing

Simultaneous or near simultaneous expansion of the rib cage and abdomen during inspiration.

Systole

Contraction, as in ventricular systole.

Tachycardia

Heart rate above the expected limits of the sinus rhythm for age, sleep/wake state and activity/status.

Term birth

Birth between 38 and 42 weeks after conception.

Theta EEG frequency band (theta rhythm)

Brain waves with a frequency of 4–8 Hz.

Tidal volume

The volume of air inspired or expired during breathing.

Time-domain

A continuous signal represented as a function of time.

Time-series

Values of the variable of interest for every instant of time from a prescribed starting time to a prescribed finishing time.

Tonic EMG

Baseline amplitudes of the EMG with an absence of stimulus-evoked increases.

Tracé alternant EEG pattern

Bursts of high-voltage slow waves, at times intermixed with sharp waves, alternating with periods of low-amplitude activity. This pattern is a feature of the period around term CA through about 52 weeks post-term.

Transient EEG arousal

As defined by the ASDA Atlas Task Force[1], an abrupt shift in EEG frequency which may include theta, alpha and/or other frequencies greater than 16 Hz but not spindles, lasting at least 3 s.

Transthoracic impedance

Electrical impedance associated with passing an AC current through the body, in this case, the thorax. Changes in breathing and cardiac cycles alter the impedance.

Vertex sharp transients

A sharp negative EEG wave that has maximal amplitude at the vertex and occurs spontaneously in sleep or in response to external stimuli. Amplitude may be as high as 250 µV.

Waveform

The shape of a wave.

REFERENCE

1. Atlas Task Force. EEG arousals: scoring rules and examples. A preliminary report from the sleep disorders Atlas Task Force of the American Sleep Disorders Association. *Sleep* 1992;15:174–84

Index

abdominal respiration, abnormal during quiet awake 81
accelerometer 29, 153
actimeter 28
  awake cf. sleep states 65
  example of activation 51
  placement on foot 52
active awake,
  crying 83
  phasic chin EMG 82
active sleep 96, 97, 153
  cf. quiet sleep 65
  in premature infant 95
activity sensors for movement 28
adjusted age 153
adult sleep stage scoring criteria 67
airflow 153
  application of electrodes for 44
  nasal 17, 23
    bandwidths used in 21
    idealized example 35
    sensors used in 21
    signals used in 21
    typical sampling rates for 20
  oral 17, 23
    bandwidths used in 21
    sensors used in 21
    signals used in 21
    typical sampling rates for 20
  sensor placement for 54
airway obstruction, arrhythmias as signs of 73
alpha rhythm 153
ALTE 156
amplification
  example of amplified signal 36
  techniques for 30
amplitude 153
analog-to-digital conversion 31, 153
apnea 153
  arousal preceding 120
  arousals and 70
  central 73, 121, 124, 125, 126, 155
  CHIME measurement of 75
  emergency procedure used in CHIME for 46
  identification of type 130
  measurement guidelines 149–150
  mixed 74, 128
  obstructive mixed 129
  obstructive sleep 74, 127, 158
  repeated 134
  rules for 149
  types of 73
architecture of sleep 109, 159
arousals 68, 153
  after central apnea 121
  after intervention 119
  classification categories 70
  definitions of 69
  hypopnea 70
  intervention 70
  on EEG 110
  post-apnea 70
  pre-apnea 70, 120
  spontaneous 70
  two scored as one 112
  unscorable 111, 113, 114, 115
arrhythmias 70, 154
  airway obstruction and 73
  asystole 123
  atrioventricular block 72
  ECG of sinus 122
  junctional escape beats 72, 123
  long QT 123
  paroxysmal atrial tachycardia 72, 123
  premature atrial beat 72, 123
  premature ventricular beat 72, 123
  respiratory sinus arrhythmia 71
  sinus bradycardia 72, 123

artifacts,
    definitions of 70
    during crying 83
    elimination of 151
    in EEG 59, 116
    in EMG 60
    movement-related 58
    pulse 61
    slow-wave 58
asynchronous respiratory effort 55
asystole 73, 123, 154
atrioventricular block 72, 154
awake state 154
    definition of 63
    maturation of physiological signals and 87

band pass filter 31, 154
band reject filter 31, 157
bandwidths used in IPSG 21
baseline drift in EEG 57
bed for sleep laboratory 40
begin study 45
behavior coding 147
bioelectric signals 154
bioelectrical potentials 154
    measurement of 22
biomedical signals, processing of 30
biopotential electrode 154
    use in measuring bioelectrical potentials 22
bipolar derivation 154
blocking 154
bodily activity summary 76
bradycardia 73, 154
    in obstructive mixed apnea 129
    in obstructive sleep apnea 127
breathing patterns 74
    paradoxical breathing 75
    periodic breathing 74
burst 154

calibration 41
    prestudy signals for 48
canthus 154
cardiac arrhythmias, see arrhythmias
cardiac definitions 70
cardiac signals, elimination of artifacts 151
cardiac summary 76
cardiorespiratory events 70
cardiorespiratory monitoring 155
cardiotachometer 155
caregiver,
    documentation by 146
    education of 139–140
central apnea 73, 124, 125, 126, 155
central hypopnea 74, 133

checklist for IPSG 141–144
CHIME,
    emergency procedure used in 46
    initiation of 15
    measurement of apnea 75
classifications, of arousals 70
CO_2,
    elimination of artifacts 151
    sensor 23, 24
        placement for 54
computer-assisted analysis 77
crying 83

decibel scale 19
delta rhythm 155
disposable nasal/oral temperature sensor 23
documentation 46, 146
dysrhythmias 71, 154

ECG 17, 155
    amplification techniques 30
    application of electrodes for 42
    arrhythmia definitions 70
    bandwidths used in 21
    filtering techniques for 31
    frequency distortion of 37
    heart rate computation and 71
    low-amplitude R-wave on 122
    movement artifact on 122
    normal 56, 122
    normal ranges of heart rate from 72
    optimal 56
    saturation distortion of 37
    sensor placement for 49
    sensors used in 21
    signals used in 21
    sinus arrhythmia 122
    testing signal quality for 45
    typical QRS recordings 71
    typical sampling rates for 20
education, of caregiver 139–140
EEG 17, 155
    activity 153
    adult cf. infants 63
    amplification techniques 30
    application of electrodes for 43
    artifacts in 59, 116
    as state scoring parameter 64
    bandwidths used in 21
    baseline drift in 57
    continuous waveforms 155
    definition of arousals from 69
    electrode positioning for ISPG 145
    frequency bands 85
    normal 86

pen blocking in 117
primary patterns in sleep states 88
pulse artifacts in 61
quiet sleep cf. active sleep 66
sensor placement for 53
sensors used in 21
signals used in 21
sleep state recognition from 64
slow-wave artifact in 58
spindle development in 64
typical sampling rates for 20
elbow covers 44
electrodes,
  application of 41
  for actimeter 43
  for airflow 44
  for ECG 42
  for EEG 43
  for EMG 43
  for EOG 43
  for movement 43
  for oximetry 42
  for position sensor 42
  for respiratory effort 42
  head wrap used in EEG 53
  movement of 51
  order of application 43
  placement for,
    actimeter 52
    airflow 54
    CO_2 54
    ECG 49
    EEG 53
    EMG 52
    EOG 52
    position 50
    pulse oximetry 50
    respiratory movement 50
  positioning for EEG 145
  protection from infants 44
  selection of 41
  typical types for IPSG 42
emergency interventions 46
EMG 17, 156
  application of electrodes for 43
  awake cf. sleep states 65
  bandwidths used in 21
  chin fluctuations during crying 83
  definition of arousals from 69
  disturbance by movement 51
  elevated tonic cf. low/absent tonic 89
  muscle artifacts in 60
  phasic chin 82
  quiet sleep cf. active sleep 66
  sensor placement for 52

sensors used in 21
signals used in 21
sucking bursts on 55
testing signal quality for 45
typical sampling rates for 20
end study 46
environment for monitoring 39
EOG 17, 156
  application of electrodes for 43
  awake cf. sleep states 64
  bandwidths used in 21
  left awake 55
  quiet sleep cf. active sleep 66
  REM in 89
  right awake 55
  sensor placement for 52
  sensors used in 21, 29
  signals used in 21
  testing signal quality for 44
  typical sampling rates for 20
epoch 156
equipment for sleep laboratory 40
explanation handout 139
eye movements, see EOG

fast activity 118
filtering 31, 156
frequency,
  distortion of ECG 37
  domains, 20
  EEG bands 85
  range 156

gain 156
gastric acid reflux 29
gastroesophageal reflux 156
glass pH electrode 30
gold electrodes 22

head wrap used in EEG sensor placement 53
heart rate 156
  computation of 71
  ECG and 71
  normal ranges of 71, 72
hemoglobin oxygen saturation 27, 156
high-pass filter 156
historical review of IPSG 15
hypercapnia 156
hypnogram 76, 137
hypopnea 131
  arousals 70
  central 74, 133
  measurement guidelines 149–150
  obstructive 74, 132, 133
  rules for 150

idiopathic apparent life-threatening event of infancy
   156
impedance 156
indeterminate sleep state 98, 100, 156
inductance plethysmography 20, 26, 157
   application of electrodes for 42
   bandwidths used in 21
   sensors used in 21
   signals used in 21
inpatient cf. outpatient monitoring 39
International 10–20 system 145, 157
interventions 46
   arousal after 119
   in emergency 46
IPSG,
   beginning of study 45
   cardiorespiratory events and 70
   checklist for 141–144
   example of report sheet 136
   historical review 15
   inpatient cf. outpatient monitoring 39
   measurement modification of international 10–20
system for 145
   physiological signal measurement for 19–37
   recording procedures for 39–61
   reliability of 66
   reports 76
   scoring procedures 63–137
   sensors and bandwidths used in 21
   sleep architecture 109
   typical sampling rates for 20
ISPG, explanation handout 139

junctional escape beats 72, 123

K-complex 157

laboratory, see sleep laboratory
lighting for sleep laboratory 40
lights out, see begin study
liquid metal strain gauge 25
long QT 123, 158
   SIDS and 72, 73
low-pass filter 157

maturation of physiological signals 87
mercury strain gauge 157
mercury switch 28
mixed apnea 74, 128
modification of international 10–20 system for IPSG
   145
monitoring,
   duration of 39
   environment for 39
   inpatient cf. outpatient 39

motion (breathing),
   artifacts 22, 157
   bandwidths used in 21
   effect on pulse oximetry 27
   sensors used in 21
   signals used in 21
   typical sampling rates for 20
movement,
   actimeter indicators 56
   activity sensors for 28
   application of electrodes for 43
   artifacts related to 58
   awake cf. sleep states 65
   body 17
   effect on EMG 51
   identification 90
   indicators of 90
   placement of actimeter for 52
   quiet sleep cf. active sleep 66
   sensors used in detecting 36
   sleep 17
   testing signal quality for 45
muscle artifacts 60

nasal airflow, see airflow
No-No's 44
nocturnal sleep 157
noise 157
   filtering techniques for 31
   measurement as time series 19
notch filter 31, 157
NREM sleep 157
Nyquist criteria 157

obstruction, partial 74
obstructive mixed apnea 129
obstructive sleep apnea 74, 127, 158
obstructive sleep hypopnea 74, 132, 133
offset 31, 158
oral airflow, see airflow
out-of-phase breathing 75, 126, 127, 135, 158
outpatient cf. inpatient monitoring 39
oximetry, see pulse oximetry
oxygen, hemoglobin saturation with 27, 156
oxygen saturation 75
oxygen saturation summary 76

P–R interval 160
paradoxical breathing 75, 126, 127, 135, 158
paroxysmal atrial tachycardia 72, 123, 158
pass frequencies 31
pen blocking 117
periodic breathing 74, 134
pH sensor 29
physiological signals 19

maturation of 87
measurement for IPSG 19–37
platinum electrodes 22
pneumogram 16, 158
position 17
    application of electrodes for 42
    electrode security and 44
    sensor output 56
    sensor placement for 50
    testing signal quality for 45
premature atrial contractions 72, 123, 158
premature ventricular contractions 72, 123, 158
prematurity and apnea 73
problem waveform recognition 45
processing of biomedical signals 30
prolonged Q–T interval 72, 73, 123, 158
pulse artifacts 61
pulse oximetry 17, 27, 158
    application of electrodes for 42
    movement and 27, 28
    sensor placement for 50
    typical sampling rates for 20

QRS complex,
    typical recordings 71
    unusual 73
QT, long, 72, 73, 123, 158
quality testing of signal 44
quality review 148
quiet awake, with irregular abdominal respiration 81
quiet sleep 99, 158
    arousals in 69
    cf. active sleep 65
    in premature infant 91, 92, 93, 94

R–R interval 159
recording,
    montage selection for in sleep laboratory 40, 41
    procedures for IPSG 39–61
reject frequencies 31
reliability of IPSG 66
REM stage sleep 108, 158
    awake cf. sleep states 64
    in left EOG 89
    in right EOG 89
    in young children 15
repeated apnea 134
report sheet for IPSG 136
resistance 159
respiratory effort 17, 159
    awake cf. sleep states 65
    quiet sleep cf. active sleep 66
    see also inductance plethysmography
    synchronous cf. asynchronous 55
    testing signal quality for 45

respiratory events 73
respiratory motion 17
    sensor placement for 50
respiratory pause 159
respiratory rate, regular/irregular calculation 89
respiratory signals, measurement of 23
respiratory sinus arrhythmia 71, 159
respiratory summary 76
rolling eye movements 159

sampling rates typical of IPSG 20
saturation 159
    distortion of ECG 37
scoring,
    adult sleep stage criteria 67
    at 3 months 68
    at 6 months 68
    CHIME criteria 67
    computer-assisted analysis 77
    definitions 69
    from EEG 64
    of arousals 69
    procedures for 63–137
    reliability of sleep state coding 66
    rules for 69
    sleep state recognition 63
    smoothing of results 68
    wake state recognition 63
sensors,
    order for application 43
    see also electrodes
    types used in IPSG 21
    used in IPSG 21
SIDS 162
    links with sleep state 15
    long QT and 72, 73
signal-to-noise ratio 19, 159
signals,
    biomedical 19
    continuous cf. sampled 34
    measurement as time series 19
    processing of biomedical signals 30
    quality testing 44
    sampled 19
    sensors used in IPSG 21
silver/silver chloride electrode 22, 159
sinus bradycardia 72, 123
    in obstructive mixed apnea 129
    in obstructive sleep apnea 127
sinus rhythm 159
sleep architecture 109, 159
sleep hypnogram 76
sleep laboratory
    preparation of,
        calibration 41

electrode selection 41
   equipment set-up 40
   recording montage selection 40
   room set-up 40
  requirements for 40
sleep position 17
sleep spindles 160
  development of 64, 85
sleep state 160
  arousal classification with 70
  arousals during 68
  determination of 65, 66
  identification 63
  maturation of physiological signals and 87
  primary EEG patterns for 88
  quiet sleep cf. active sleep 65
  recognition of 63, 64, 65
  reliability of coding 66
  scoring criteria for 67, 68
  scoring methods at 3 months 68
  scoring methods at 6 months 68
  smoothing of results 68, 137
sleep study 16
sleep summary 76
slow eye movements 159
slow-wave artifact 58
smoothing 68, 137
source impedance 22, 160
spindle development 64, 85
staffing 39

stage 1 sleep 101, 160
stage 2 sleep 102, 103, 104, 160
stage 3 sleep 105, 106, 160
stage 4 sleep 107, 160
stage REM sleep 108
sucking bursts on EMG 55
synchronous respiratory effort 55, 160

tachycardia 160
temperature for sleep laboratory 40
thermistors 23
theta rhythm 160
tidal volume 160
time-domain 20, 160
time-series 160
transition state, wake to sleep 84
transthoracic impedance 24, 161
  bandwidths used in 21
  sensors used in 21
  signals used in 21

vertex sharp transients 161

wake state,
  definitions of 69
  recognition of 63
wave signals 34
waveforms 161
  problem recognition 45